E. P. M. Woollacott
2013

ROBERT N. BUTLER, MD

ROBERT N. BUTLER, MD

Visionary of Healthy Aging

W. ANDREW ACHENBAUM

Columbia University Press

New York

Columbia University Press
Publishers Since 1893
New York   Chichester, West Sussex
cup.columbia.edu
Copyright © 2013 Columbia University Press
All rights reserved

Library of Congress Cataloging-in-Publication Data

Achenbaum, W. Andrew.
    Robert N. Butler, MD : visionary of healthy aging / W. Andrew Achenbaum.
        pages   cm
    Includes bibliographical references and index.
    ISBN 978-0-231-16442-9 (cloth : alk. paper) — ISBN 978-0-231-53532-8 (e-book)
    1. Butler, Robert N., 1927–2010.   2. Gerontologists—United States—
Biography.   3. Gerontology—United States.   I. Title.

    HQ1064.U5B8733 2013
    305.26092—dc23
    [B]

                                                    2012048642

Columbia University Press books are printed on permanent
and durable acid-free paper.
This book is printed on paper with recycled content.
Printed in the United States of America
c 10 9 8 7 6 5 4 3 2 1

Cover design by Jordan Wannemacher
Cover image by Robert Caplin, courtesy of the *New York Times*/Redux

References to websites (URLs) were accurate at the time of writing. Neither the
author nor Columbia University Press is responsible for URLs that may have
expired or changed since the manuscript was prepared.

*To Robert N. Butler's daughters
—Cynthia, Carole, Christine, and Alexandra—
and to his grandchildren and great-grandchildren*

And in memory of Myrna I. Lewis (1938–2005)

CONTENTS

PREFACE

Robert Neil Butler, MD

(January 21, 1927–July 4, 2010)

Dr. Robert N. Butler became the "Visionary of Healthy Aging" here and abroad by dint of his five decades of groundbreaking research, influential writing, prudent institution building, and diligent networking. He helped to transform the study of aging from a marginal specialty into an intellectually vibrant field of inquiry. Gerontology now attracts the attention of renowned scholars, emerging professionals, students, and other experts who are determined to understand the secrets of longevity and healthy aging. Butler designed, underwrote, and conveyed perspectives on aging rigorous enough to impress scientific peers and practical enough to sway policy makers and politicians. A psychiatrist and geriatrician, Butler also initiated changes in the training of physicians and other health professionals on how to care for the elderly. All this had a profound impact on altering the lay public's images of the aged: Butler gave people reason to question stereotypes that demeaned late life and cause to focus on healthy, productive aging.

With Butler's death a formative chapter in the history of gerontology and geriatrics ended: we are unlikely to see in our lifetimes anyone so adept at generating, championing, and communicating issues in aging. Butler exemplified the importance of interdisciplinarity in advancing research, education, and policy making in gerontological practices. Geriatrics, he stressed, was more than a medical specialty that complemented family medicine; it offered a team approach to addressing older people's resources and resilience while attending to diseases and challenges of late life.

No contemporary gerontologist or geriatrician moved as deftly as Butler from one domain of American life to another. He and his ideas became a significant presence in medical schools and higher education, the media, hospitals and laboratories, literary and cultural organizations, foundations, and government agencies. He left an ambitious agenda for future work in geriatrics and gerontology. Those who continue to work in these and related fields would do well to capitalize on three of Butler's remarkable strengths: (1) his dogged determination to stimulate and refine scientific investigations concerning various dimensions of human aging, (2) his gifts for conveying images to the public that illuminate the meanings and experiences of late life, and (3) his capacity for mentoring, in addition to his remarkable generosity to those who aspired to improve the quality of late life.

Butler was an idea broker. In his twenties, when he was a fledgling investigator and physician, he saw potential for personal growth among people advancing in years. Whereas most physicians and clinicians in the 1950s and 1960s focused on aging as a disease-ridden period of decline, he extolled later years' positive qualities. Eager to broaden and clarify scientific modes of gerontology, Butler devoted his career to promoting means to enhance older people's health, esteem, and social roles. He gleefully crossed disciplinary frontiers to challenge and uproot disparaging views of human aging; he endeavored to replace stereotypes with images that accorded older individuals everywhere dignity and respect.

Butler envisioned a new millennium that held unprecedented opportunities for productive aging. "Many of our economic, political, ethical, health, and other institutions, such as education and work life, have been *rendered obsolete* by the added years of life for so many citizens," he proclaimed in the *Longevity Revolution* (2008:17). In the midst of the modern Longevity Revolution, which was transforming individual ways of growing older and vectors of societal aging, healthy elders could and should use their talents and experiences to benefit youth. Commentators in the United States and abroad saluted Butler's vision. "No one did more to change society's perceptions of ageing and the aged than Robert Butler," declared the obituary writer of the *Guardian* in Britain (Carlson, 2010), "because his greatest achievement was in changing the attitude that obsolescence was the inevitable product of the ageing process."

Butler the idea broker also proved to be a masterful wordsmith. Over the course of his career, Butler coined many words and phrases now used to describe the meanings and conditions of being older. For instance, as a newly minted psychiatrist, he developed the concept of the "life review," a technique to assist elderly men and women grappling with issues still unresolved from earlier in their lives as they came to face death's inevitability. Therapists fifty years later still use this technique to encourage clients to journal their journey of life. And, as we shall see in chapter 1, Butler himself revisited his ideas about life review in his last weeks.

In his mid-fifties Butler introduced the idea of "productive aging" to embrace the contributions elders made in their households, volunteer activities, and late-life careers. Others, taking cues from him, added "successful," "vital," "conscious," and "positive" aging to the repertoire. Such themes remain prominent in popular books, news reports, media releases, and research articles. They all underscore positive aspects of growing older.

Well past normal retirement age, Butler sought to broaden the range and focus of aging studies. The consequences of demographic shifts associated with the Longevity Revolution, he believed, required scientists to develop fresh scientific constructs for studying societal aging and to create new institutional arrangements and normative patterns to accommodate individuals benefiting from extended years of maturation. Summing up a rich career of exchanges with other idea brokers, he mapped out the parameters of what he called the "New Gerontology" in *The Longevity Revolution*, articulating a bold model with which to analyze and harvest the fruits of extra years. While disappointed by the poor receptivity to his ideas, he nonetheless exuded his hallmark self-confidence as he insisted that he was on the right track.

There were frustrations other than intellectual disappointments. Butler well understood that ignorance, prejudice, and stereotypes clouded the vision of vital, productive, fruitful aging that he wished to promulgate. The mistreatment of older patients in health-care facilities and the neglect of geriatrics by the medical establishment had begun to anger him while he was still an intern. Butler chastised colleagues for presuming that the depressed outlook and physical impairments common among the institutionalized aged represented the "normal" profile of older Americans. Butler gave the odious prejudice a name: in 1968 he coined the term "ageism" as an analog to "racism" and "sexism." *Ageism* quickly entered everyday parlance. Ageism undermines the value and status of elderly men and women in virtually every sector of American life—notably education, health care, the labor market, and the media—and remains there to this day.

In late life Butler concluded that ageism was even more pernicious and invidious than he initially had realized. In "Combatting Ageism: A Matter of Human and Civil Rights," his introduction to a report on *Ageism in America* (2006:1), Butler opined that

> the status of older persons and our attitudes toward them are not only rooted in historic and economic circumstances. They also derive from deeply held human concerns and fears about the vulnerability inherent in the later years of life. . . . Older people are still being rendered invisible. Instances of this invisibility occurred in the horrific aftermath of Hurricane Katrina when a person's class (impoverished) and race (black) were dominating factors in survival. Older persons in their own homes and in nursing homes were often abandoned.

Butler now called ageism a disease, a morbid fear of decline and death that crippled individuals.

Outrage at the disregard and devaluation of older persons impelled him to write *Why Survive? Being Old in America* (1975b), which won a Pulitzer Prize. "When we talk about old age, each of us is talking about his or her own future," Butler wrote. "We must ask ourselves if we are willing to settle for mere survival when so much more is possible." From a man usually guarded about expressing feelings, this sentence reveals much about Robert Butler and his raison d'être: the visionary of healthy aging rarely hesitated to forcefully challenge conventional wisdom about aging when he felt it was wrong or misguided.

Nor did Butler accept "mere survival" as the baseline for living, despite moments in own his life history that tested his resilience and perseverance. The Great Depression shaped his childhood, exposing him to poverty and loss, material and familial. Grieving the death of his beloved wife, Myrna Lewis, for the rest of his days, he nonetheless remained open to new love. On top of his strenuous writing and travel schedules, he found time to grant interviews and to support diverse cultural and political causes. Butler invariably accentuated the positive, quick to note progress made. He championed causes for older Americans with unrelenting optimism. Sometimes such an ebullient outlook blinded him to inconvenient truths in the marketplace of ideas and in his dealings with others.

Appointed in 1976 by President Gerald Ford to be the first director of the National Institute on Aging (NIA), Butler took daring, sometimes controversial, steps: he made research on Alzheimer's disease a priority at NIA instead of earmarking incremental resources into basic biomedical mechanisms and processes of aging. After he moved to Mount Sinai Medical Center in New York to establish the country's first geriatrics department, federal and local cost-cutting measures made it difficult for him to secure budget increases for elder care. That he flourished so long in an era of superspecialization and zero-sum academic politics attests to Butler's savvy and leadership style. After initially playing to his strengths in basic sciences at the International Longevity Center, he delved heavily into economics and ethics, two areas where he was not trained.

The outpouring of affection in obituaries in the United States and around the world demonstrates the respect and admiration bestowed on Robert Butler. According to Catherine Mayer (2010), who interviewed him for *Time* a few weeks before his death, "he proved a role model, right until the end, as he was energetic and effective." Christine Cassel, MD, president of the American Board of Internal Medicine, remembered her mentor this way: "Bob Butler [had] an amazing ability to keep both engaging personal stories and attention-grabbing statistics on the tip of his tongue. . . . For those of us who watched his effective presentations, these speeches were themselves worthy objects of study. We realized that carrying the baton he handed to us required understanding the skills of persuasion just as much as the skills of being a good geriatric clinician or researcher" (Cassel, 2010).

Butler was a can-do, go-to guy, at once a cheerleader and a taskmaster who expected the best from others and certainly nothing less from himself. He was a loyal friend who routinely checked up on college roommates. Butler traveled easily in the rarified circuit between Washington and New York. Although received royally abroad, he remained hospitable to strangers, unfailingly courteous to all.

In November 2009 Robert Butler showed me a draft of a memoir he said that he had written for his four daughters and grandchildren. Having known Butler for thirty years, I suspected that he intended to publish what he had written. When I told him bluntly that the text needed a lot of work, he invited me to edit it. I replied that I preferred to write his biography. He worried that my rendition would be too flattering; I assured him that that would not be an issue.

I worked with Bob on this book until he died. Besides sharing his love of history and ideas, I knew the names of most of his friends, and I interviewed key colleagues in geriatrics and gerontology. I enjoyed listening to him ruminate about science and culture, revise his action plan for what he absolutely had to accomplish within the next five years, and express his love for and pride in his daughters. Two weeks after his death, to honor one of Butler's last intentions, I traveled with three of his daughters and his dear friend on an itinerary he had planned—to Vineland, New Jersey, where Bob spent his early years, and to Rehoboth Beach, Delaware, where the family usually vacationed in August.

My main purpose in writing *Robert N. Butler, MD: Visionary of Healthy Aging* has been to interpret how this éminence grise helped to shape the history of gerontology and geriatrics in the United States during a critical period of development. Butler's life personified the ripening of the greatest human possibilities into advanced age. His life work refracted and reflected trends in American medical, policy, political, gerontological, and geriatric history during the last half-century. Because his public record is so rich, I chose not to quote directly from his memoir: the document clearly is a work in progress, and I want to respect Dr. Butler's right to privacy. That said, I must quickly add that his prodigious output made it easy to find in print ideas often fragmented in his unfinished manuscript.

I have concentrated in this book on Butler's evolving ideas about aging and his professional modus operandi, which permeate the study and practice of gerontology and geriatrics today and in the future. There is a need for a work that critically assesses the hurdles he faced. Butler was a Renaissance man whose ideas will foreshadow developments for some time to come. At the same time I hope that it will be instructive for baby boomers and those entering the field to come to terms with the historical vectors that frustrated him and kept him from completing his agenda.

With the graying of the baby boomer generation, the coming of age inevitably will have as great an impact on public discourse and societal institutions as did the Civil Rights movement and the feminist revolution, in which boomers participated as youth. What we have learned and distilled since World War II about age and aging should impel thoughtful readers and activists to build on Butler's legacy and, ideally, go farther than he did in integrating gerontological research, geriatric care, age-based coalitions, and generational politics into other domains of life. Butler, working at the vanguard of the new gerontology, sought to expand intellectual horizons and social mores. He had faith in the leaders of academic gerontology and medical centers, but the insularity of many coworkers dismayed him. Ageism remains endemic. These are some of the reasons why Butler did not totally succeed in creating a bold vision of aging America that captured the imaginations of scientific communities, lawmakers, and the public.

I wish to explicate the relevance of Butler's brilliant exploration of the meanings and experiences of growing older and societal aging over the past half-century. This vision not only illuminates contemporary age-groups and institutions, but it will be the touchstone for future developments. This book builds on an emerging literature on developments in the field of aging as well as cultural and social histories of postwar America. I have rethought and recast ideas that I presented in *Crossing Frontiers: Gerontology Emerges as a Science* (Achenbaum, 1995). I have updated the main lines of Butler's own unedited bio-sketch that he contributed to *Profiles in Gerontology: A Biographical Dictionary* (Achenbaum & Albert, 1995). Butler's family and friends have been very supportive, especially after Bob's death, but I alone bear responsibility for what follows. As Butler would have wished, I have composed a comprehensive, sometimes critical interpretation of a trailblazer who contributed much to improve the well-being of all who are or will become elders in postwar America, a critical period of U.S. cultural and social history.

ACKNOWLEDGMENTS

This book began as a joint venture between the late Robert N. Butler and me. I interviewed Dr. Butler on four separate occasions early in 2010 and corresponded with him by phone and e-mail until his sudden death. Three of his daughters—Alexandra, Chris, and Cindy—and one of his granddaughters (Corinne) gave me insights, personal and professional, into a man they adored. It is fitting to dedicate this volume to them. I also want to thank Herta Gordon, who enriched Bob's life, for her support and perspectives.

Friends were tremendous help. I owe my greatest debt to Rick Moody, who willingly interrupted our collaborative efforts on two other books so that I could undertake this project in a timely manner. Having worked closely with Butler for more than three decades, Rick provided a reading of the first draft of the manuscript that proved enormously helpful. He also offered tough constructive criticism when he felt that I needed it. Tom Cole greatly improved the first chapter. Linda Fried and Jack Rowe made the initial pitch to Columbia University Press. Morriseen Barmore, Butler's assistant, and our mutual friend Barbara Greenberg supplied hard-to-find materials. Wyneth Carter Achenbaum, my sister-in-law, did invaluable genealogical searches. I also benefited from conversations and friends in U.S. gerontological and geriatric circles—especially Bob Atchley, the late Bob Binstock, Tuck Finch, Bob Kastenbaum, and "Fox" Wetle.

I wrote much of this manuscript while serving as a visiting chair in gerontology at St. Thomas University in Fredericton, New Brunswick. There Gary Kenyon, Bill Randall, and Deb van den Hoonaard provided terrific support; Janice Ryan did a superb job of editing an early draft. Stephen Katz arranged for talks at Trent University and the University of Toronto, generously offering his perspective. Thanks to my colleagues at the University of Houston and the Institute for Spirituality and Health, I had the time necessary to revise my work. Maria von Furstenberg, Claire Poff, and Nicole Kurtz helped to organize citations. Colleagues in the Department of Geriatric and Palliative Care Medicine, University of Texas Medical School Houston, gave me valuable feedback, especially Carmel Dyer and Sharon Ostwald. I found it useful to bounce ideas off Earl Shelp, an associate at Interfaith Care Partners.

At Columbia University Press, Jennifer Perillo has been an enthusiastic and discerning editor. I have also benefited from working with Stephen Wesley, Kathryn Jorge, Emily Loeb, Anita O'Brien, and Pat Perrier.

ROBERT N. BUTLER, MD

one
LIFE REVIEW

"Life review" has become a standard method of working with older people in clinical settings and adult learning centers. Life review gives older people an opportunity to arrange the threads of their biographies. They can review afresh both the primary and dystonic motifs that become manifest in the process. Ideally, life review—rarely a one-time exercise— prepares subjects to face finitude with equanimity, possibly to tie up loose ends in representations of self and relationships with others.

I start with life review because Butler, at age thirty-six, stressed its value for treating the aged—even those abandoned in nursing homes. His ideas and methods quickly gained wide usage for younger persons as well. He himself engaged in life reviews of his own at several junctures, includ- ing the very end of his life. Life review thus affords us a synoptic aperçu into Butler and his ideas as he aged.

※ ※ ※ ※ ※

Early in his scientific career Butler fired gerontological imaginations with a path-breaking article, "The Life Review: An Interpretation of Reminiscence in the Aged" (1963b). This article questioned whether late life was invariably a period of deterioration and loss. Psychiatrists and other health-care professionals, according to Butler, too often presumed that mental, physical, and socioeconomic decline determined experiences and meanings associated with advancing years. "It is fair to say that the major portion of gerontological literature throughout the country is concerned almost enthusiastically with measuring decline in various cognitive, perceptual, and psychomotor functions" (Neugarten, 1968). Butler thought otherwise, based on his talking with elders residing both independently and institutionally. Convinced that his research into late-life mental health corroborated his clinical experiences, two related areas in which few other scientists did work, he set out to overturn conventional wisdom by interpreting late-life reminiscences as a normal, integral activity. Doing life review made Butler certain that there was far more to aging than declining.

The publication and dissemination of "The Life Review" greatly affected many mental-health workers after 1963. "I was then a very junior social worker on the staff of a home for the aged," recalled gerontologist Rose Dobrof. "The Butler paper came out and was read and talked about and our world changed." Dobrof added, "In a profound sense, Butler's writings liberated both the old and the nurses, doctors and social workers; the old were free to remember, to regret, to look reflectively at the past and try to understand it. And we were free to listen and treat rememberers and remembrances with the respect they deserved, instead of trivializing them by diversion to a bingo game" (1984:xvii–xviii).

People in the field increasingly embraced Butler's presentation of what late-life remembrances signified. Accepting Butler's argument meant that reminiscing would no longer be viewed as "pathology—regression to the dependency of the child, denial of the passage of time, and the reality of the present, or evidence of organic impairment of the intellect" (Dobrof, 1984:xviii). Changing entrenched professional views of reminiscences was going to take time, however.

Health-care professionals in postwar America mainly concentrated on deficits accumulated with advancing age, Butler contended. Most of his peers underestimated—indeed, missed altogether—older people's ongoing capacity to learn and to grow. His contemporaries generally were not interested in identifying, measuring, and evaluating positive attributes of growing older; they did not look for assets and advantages that accrued over time because they reckoned that there was little to find. Deeply held biases against age, according to Butler, caused scientists and clinicians to misinterpret elders' reminiscences. For instance, Dr. Theodore Lidz, an expert on schizophrenia at Yale, classified reminiscences as "memory impairments":

> Elderly people, as is well known, spend an increasing amount of time talking and thinking about the past. . . . When the future holds little, and thinking about it arouses thoughts of death, interest will turn regressively to earlier years. Still, in most persons who become very old, the defect is more profound. . . . This type of memory failure depends on senile changes in the brain and is perhaps the most characteristic feature of senility.
>
> (LIDZ, 1968:487)

It was such characterizations of reminiscences, expressed in scientific terms with clinical detachment, that Butler sought to overturn. To him, memory work with older patients was worth doing: through the life review a therapist might hope to sustain or restore in clients those attitudes and behaviors conducive to healthy aging. Some elderly people who uttered meaningless, garrulous sentiments reverted to childlike behavior, he recognized. In such instances reminiscences probably were manifestations of depression or some other late-life malady. Yet "hidden themes of great vintage may emerge," Butler felt, in memories shared and discussed between patients and therapists (Neugarten, 1968:496).

Embellishing this motif—with the therapeutic aim of recovering or (better yet) uncovering potentials of old age so that individuals could enjoy a ripe maturity in a manner beneficial to society—became one of the major priorities of Butler's long and distinguished career as a physician, research scientist, medical educator, policy analyst, and public intellectual in the United States and abroad. It sustained an even bolder aim. For nearly six decades he formulated positive images of age as he attacked stereotypic ones. In this context the asset-based approach to aging in "The Life Review," now widely accepted among practitioners working with elders, can be seen at its outset as a harbinger of things to come.

Butler initially described "The Life Review" as an *interpretation*, not a scientific theory. The concept's scope and usefulness would evolve, he reckoned, as life review's value as an integrative psychological process was debated and modified. The apposition of "life review" to "reminiscence" in the paper's full title, however, did not mean that he considered these key words to be equivalents (Woodward, 1997). Life reviews might stimulate personal insights that elders preferred to keep private, whereas reminiscences generally are shared. Life reviews analyze an individual's entire life, whereas reminiscences usually evoke moods surrounding particular moments. Here is Butler's definition of life review in 1963:

> I conceive of the life review as a naturally occurring, universal mental process characterized by the progressive return to consciousness of past experiences, and, particularly, the resurgence of unresolved conflicts; simultaneously, and normally, these revived experiences and conflicts can be surveyed and reintegrated. Presumably this process is prompted by the realization of approaching dissolution and death, and the inability to maintain one's sense of personal invulnerability. It is further shaped by contemporaneous experiences and by the life-long unfolding of character.
>
> (NEUGARTEN, 1968:487)

To Butler, life review entailed critical analyses that stimulated ubiquitous, natural, and normal mental processes in assessing the quality of life. The imaginations and memories of older people brought to surface materials from their unconscious. Free association, recall, and assessment, he argued, ideally would illuminate "progressive" steps for older persons to take as they tackled two ultimate challenges: (1) addressing issues unresolved from earlier in their life histories and (2) preparing for death.

Acknowledging vulnerability and coming to terms with dying and death surely were life events likely to trigger life reviews. The unfolding process could take many turns, ranging from redemptive to self-defeating. Particularly in late life, mourning could induce guilt or inspire gratitude for life's gifts; grieving losses might prompt restitutions or kindle a desire to leave a legacy (Kaminsky, 1984:12–13). A wide array of metaphors of self emerged from life review.

The vicissitudes of life, observed Butler, provoked diverse responses. Life review hopefully helped elders to revive memories that, when integrated with how they assessed their vulnerability, engendered "candor, serenity, and wisdom." Engaging in the process did not always yield positive results, however. Struggling to work through long-standing, unresolved conflicts was risky business. So was piecing together seemingly irreconcilable facets of one's life, especially if the client were unaccustomed to "intrepid exploring" (Lee, 2010:18). Some elders became threatened by discoveries that undercut changes in equanimity, or they became distracted when focusing on past events.

An important, lasting message in Butler's original formulation of "The Life Review" is his unequivocal affirmation that the process he had created often had negative outcomes. Attempts to make sense of the past, he wrote, could spark feelings of regret, anxiety, despair, and depression, or aggravate neuroses. Life review might reinforce false illusions of self. "Although a favorable, constructive, and positive end result may be enhanced by favorable environmental circumstances, such as comparative freedom from crises and losses, it is more likely that successful reorganization is a function of personality—in particular, such vaguely defined features of the personality as flexibility, resilience, and self-awareness" (Neugarten, 1968:490).

Butler never claimed to have invented the concept of life review. In fact his 1963 paper included three historical references to late-life reminiscing: one ambiguous, one flattering, and one dismaying, each drawn from different historical periods. He first invoked lines from Aristotle's *Rhetoric*: "[Elders] live by memory rather than hope, for what is left to them of life is but little compared to the long past. This, again, is the cause of their loquacity. They are constantly talking of the past, because they enjoy remembering." The passage was ambiguous. Did elders in ancient Greece, like us, try to deny death by looking backwards? Or, did talking about the past help them savor whatever time remained to them? The second allusion, from the eighteenth-century English poet and hymn composer William Cowper, in contrast, was more upbeat: he praised "mem'ry's pointing wand, that calls the past to our exact review." Finally, in quoting Somerset Maugham (1874–1965), Butler presaged the dark shadow of life review: Maugham at age eighty-five declared that "what makes old age hard to bear is not a failing of one's faculties, mental and physical, but the burden of one's memories" (Neugarten, 1968:486).

Literary and historical references rarely are found in scientific papers, but "Butler elevates literature to the status of truth in the scientific sense" (Woodward, 1986:146). The humanities and arts were not ornamental; to him, they served to ground clinical findings. Elsewhere, in linking the life-review process to thoughts about death, Butler referred to the matador's "moment of truth" during the faena; he then punctuated his notion of the life review as a Janus-like process by mentioning Lot and Orpheus. Furthermore, he praised Ingmar Bergman's *Wild Strawberries* (1957) as "a beautiful example of the constructive aspects of the life review" (Neugarten, 1968:488, 490).

That said, the 1963 interpretation rested on his earlier work as well as the best available psychological theories of aging and prototypes of life review that emerged as part of intensive psychotherapeutic relationships. To document deleterious reactions to life review associated with isolation, loneliness, and death, Butler cited studies by Walter Cannon, Frieda Fromm-Reichmann, Curt Richter, and Otto Will, among others, whose work was respected by gerontologists. He then moved to actual case studies of "manifestations of the life review." He concluded his 1963 article by citing Erik Erikson's epigenetic model, which mapped out successive stages of identity over the course of human development. Butler asserted that "the entire life cycle cannot be comprehended without inclusion of the psychology of the aged" (Neugarten, 1968:488, 496).

After disclosing his wide-ranging sources of inspiration, Butler took credit for some clinical observations about the positive value of reminiscences; he also acknowledged his role in developing techniques to prompt elders to recapture meaning in their lives. Life review, he noted, was not orderly: "Although the process is active, not static, the content of one's life usually unfolds slowly; the process may not be completed prior to death" (Neugarten, 1968:488). It requires time, he realized, for individuals to synthesize random musings about their life histories into a cogent narrative. Far from discounting reminiscences as signs of "psychological dysfunction," Butler wanted to help elders make stories out of their lives' messiness by letting the past inform current challenges and contingencies.

Butler deliberately included in his subject pool aged patients in hospitals and other institutional settings; he recognized life review's efficacy among lonely, confined elders. Extrapolating from this idea, subsequent researchers attested that reminiscing might mitigate incipient dementia (Webster, Bohlmeijer, & Westerhof, 2010). Older people were better off, suggested Butler, if they learned to contemplate and prepare for what lay ahead. Life review offered elders a perspective on ways in which past experiences had brought them to their present situation. (Mental) health professionals, he lamented, generally overlooked their older clients' need to look both backward and forward. "Younger therapists especially, working with the elderly, find great difficulties in listening," Butler observed in 1963, because clinicians were not trained to heed what older people were saying (Neugarten, 1968:486). His approach to reminiscences in "The Life Review," extending earlier work, presented clinicians with a counterintuitive way of interpreting how patients assess their accomplishments, deal with unfinished business, and plan legacies as they prepare to die (Butler, 1961).

MODIFICATIONS TO THE ORIGINAL FORMULATION OF LIFE REVIEW

Robert Butler periodically revisited his initial formulations concerning the purposes and value of life review. Interactions with patients (mostly healthy older adults in the Washington, D.C., area during the 1950s and 1960s) facilitated his evaluations. "Hearing them talk about their lives, I was so struck by the importance of it—the energy, the value, the effort to come to terms with their lives, to think about reconciling with others," he recalled. "It was just a knock-out" (Wood, 2008). By 1974 he was asserting that life review fostered successful aging (Butler, 1974). Meanwhile, he devised a questionnaire to study creativity over the life course; among the notables interviewed in these unguided autobiographies was behaviorist B. F. Skinner (Kleyman, 2011). During the 1976 bicentennial celebrations, as part of the Smithsonian Institution's oral history project, he collaborated with anthropologists Margaret Mead and Wilton Dillon to record for posterity the experiences and memories of ordinary people. Butler told me that visitors from all across the nation lined up to share their stories at tables that the trio set up on the Mall.

To underscore his contention that life review took many forms, Butler proposed "several methods of evoking memory in older persons that are useful and often enjoyable to them" (Lewis & Butler, 1974:166). He gave examples in an article entitled "Life-Review Therapy: Putting Memories to Work in Individual and Group Psychotherapy," coauthored with social worker and psychotherapist Myrna I. Lewis, who shortly became his second wife and the love of his life. The pair recommended seven approaches: (1) embarking on written or taped autobiographies; (2) making pilgrimages to the locations of one's birth, childhood, youth, or young adulthood; (3) attending family or school reunions; (4) taking an interest in genealogy; (5) preserving scrapbooks, photo albums, old letters, and other memorabilia; (6) summing up the meaning of one's life work; and (7) preserving ethnic identity. Note the shift in the presentation of what prompts life review: Butler now was declaring that all sorts of memories (including ones not directly linked to the proximity of death) could trigger reminiscences useful in the task of coming to terms with the meanings of one's life.

Other changes also occurred, even in psychotherapeutic settings where life reviews take place. Beginning in 1970 Lewis and Butler started to experiment with *group* psychotherapy. They conducted sessions with participants as young as age fifteen. The presence of youth altered the milieu in which older people focused on reminiscences. "The elderly often assume an active learning as well as a teaching role," reported the co-therapists. "Groups are especially useful in decreasing the sense of isolation and uselessness felt by many elderly persons" (Lewis & Butler, 1974:173).

During this period Butler also developed a *Life-Review Interview Manual* with questions intended to bring to the forefront distinctive features of individuals' life histories concerning child-rearing, marriage, and careers. Besides furnishing basic biographical details, older adults were asked to flesh out what made some of their friendships special. They were invited to talk about persons who were important in their lives. Additional questions sought to explore what people recalled about situations during the Great Depression and World War II that they had endured with others. Still other inquiries gauged how elders assessed their current circumstances (Butler, 2002b; Kleyman, 2011).

Like facets of a widening gyre, the items in Butler's *Life-Review Interview Manual* were designed to stimulate people's interest in narrating their lives. In the 1970s neither Butler nor Lewis was consistent in differentiating between retrieving memories and engaging in life review. This imprecision provoked criticism. According to William Randall and Elizabeth McKim, "the difference between retrieving our memory and reviewing our life is the difference between a store-wide inventory of the stock on the shelves and audit of the books. . . . such a tallying clearly has its place, yet there is always more material tucked away in memory than meets the conscious mind" (2008:171). Life review, suggest Randall and McKim, empowers willing individuals to move from what they *do* remember to what they *can* remember in order to vivify hidden feelings.

Nor did the psychotherapeutic interventions and programmed activities recommended by Butler and Lewis exhaust options for embarking on this exercise. The pair recognized that elders could utilize various approaches to composing life reviews. James Birren, who was Butler's professional colleague of longest standing, independently collaborated over the years with students and associates at the University of Southern California to develop techniques for constructing guided autobiographies (Birren & Deutchman, 1991). Memoirs, a genre that dated back at least to St. Augustine's *Confessions*, offered another model conducive to doing life review. In papers and speeches Butler referred to introspective struggles manifest in modern-day memoirs, such as Robert McNamara's *The Tragedy and Lessons of Vietnam* (1995) and Larry McMurty's *Roads: Driving America's Great Highways* (2000). While none of these approaches "necessarily represent the unvarnished truth," Butler noted roughly four decades after beginning work on life review, reminiscence per se would not constitute "true" life review unless it entailed a critical assessment of prior events in a subject's life.

INTERDISCIPLINARY ADAPTATIONS OF THE LIFE REVIEW

As the life-review concept became more widespread, psychiatrists were not the only group to seize on its therapeutic value. Specialists and practitioners across academic disciplines and health-care professions adapted Robert Butler's interpretation and protocols for their own purposes. A few examples attest to the varied, varying uses made of life review:

• Life review has been incorporated into specific therapeutic approaches, such as cognitive-behavioral and narrative therapies. It was also used to insinuate specific positive memories that elude depressed individuals in the course of everyday activities (Bohlmeijer, Westerhof, & Emmerik de-Jong, 2008; Cappeliez, 2002; Steunenberg & Bohlmeijer, 2011). Mental-health experts compiled guidebooks and handbooks for use in practice (Haight & Haight, 2007; Kunz & Soltys, 2007; Webster & Haight, 2002).

• Social workers utilized life-review approaches in helping clients initiating or dealing (for better or worse) with matters such as the consequences of late-life divorce. Results sometimes were disappointing: "There was no evidence of life review as a common coping strategy" (Weingarten, 1988).

• Palliative-care workers developed a five-stage life review to help dying patients find "life reconciliation" as they sought to reach closure with a sense of completion (Morrow, 2009).

• Two creative groups in New York, who belonged to the Artists & Elders Project and the Teachers & Writers Collaborative, used reminiscences and life review in conducting workshops in senior centers, nursing homes, libraries, union halls, and casework agencies. Some artists conjoined life review, performances in living-history theater, and community-based social-work practices (Kaminsky, 1988:xv; Perlstein, 1988). The use of life review and reminiscence interventions was modified to reach subsets of the older population, such as gays and lesbians, rural elders, persons with chronic illness, and war veterans (Kenyon, Bohlmeijer, & Randall, 2010:275). Geriatricians, therapists, caregivers, and other professionals who refined life-review applications created institutional supports, such as organizing in 1995 the International Society for Reminiscence and Life Review.

Twenty-five years after Butler's initial presentation, life review was attracting ever wider applications and broader audiences. "There is something to this idea of reminiscence and life review that is compelling, something which is very far from being merely a form of group-work or a technique of therapy. The idea of life review is, finally, more akin to a wish, a hope, an act of the imagination itself," wrote H. R. (Rick) Moody (1988:8). He went on to observe:

> Life history activities evoke our most deeply held hopes and wishes about what the last stage of life should be. Those hopes are just that: not "facts," but a kind of myth or collective wish-fulfillment intent on transforming old age in modern society and, ultimately, offering an alternative sense of meaning in a world where the last stage of life tends to be drained of meaning altogether. This does not mean that life review is to be rejected or even demythologized. But if I am correct in my suspicion that life review is a new kind of gerontological myth, then it deserves the most serious scrutiny.
>
> (12)

Lest life review become what Moody characterized as "a kind of ersatz religion," researchers on aging mounted serious critiques.

CRITICISMS OF THE LIFE REVIEW

Criticisms were far-ranging. The conceptual foundations of Butler's original formulation and subsequent protocols for doing life reviews were challenged. Some investigators and practitioners doubted that life review was a universal process psychologically dependent, as Butler claimed, on the ego's strength as death approached. Others reported that middle-aged participants and younger ones could benefit as much from life review as elders. Gender, ethnicity, and personality, proposed a few, were better predictors than age per se in successful handling of life-review transformations (Tornstam, 2005; Webster & Haight, 2002; Woodward, 1986).

Evaluating applications at both ends of the life course, researchers questioned how, precisely, crises (such as the prospect of imminent death) impel older people into life review. Were centenarians more likely to benefit than younger participants? Assessing children's memory capacities and identities of self, in turn, invited developmental psychologists to move beyond the writings of Erik Erikson and Butler; they related life review to theories by Heinz Kohut, Margaret Mahler, and D. W. Winnicott (Disch, 1988; Kohut, 2000; Mahler, Pine, & Bergman, 1973; Winnicott, 1971).

Another line of criticism disputed the merits of unstructured approaches to life review, particularly in situations where participants were trying to retrieve important yet potentially painful memories. In working with people with serious mental illnesses, some psychologists argued that "the focus is to reduce bitterness and boredom and to stimulate the positive functions of reminiscence . . . intervention protocols must be explicit" (Bohlmeijer & Westerhof, 2010:277). Meanwhile, others were concerned that engaging in life review could prevent denial, a prime defense mechanism in late life, or temper the desire of a "golden ager" to fantasize in order to adapt to the present (Kaminsky, 1988:151).

Methodological issues were raised: How definitively could participants and observers validate memories? What was the empirical connection between life review and reminiscence? How were benefits that accrued from life review to be measured? Was life review, as social constructionists contended, "a social activity occasioned by narrative challenges rather than an outward manifestation of an internal psychodevelopmental process?" (Wallace, 1992:120).

Finally, many theorists and methodologists were keen to situate life review (as well as reminiscences, autobiographies, and memories) in new understandings of "narrative discourse," which began to transpose ways of seeing, particularly in the human sciences, during the 1980s. The paradigm shift is evident in contributions to *Aging and Biography* (1996). "In their own efforts to understand human behavior and experience," noted Dan McAdams, "many social scientists have come around to *the story* to vitalize their methods and their concepts for the study of lives." Those doing life reviews, observed investigators, appreciated the power of storytelling. "When aging adults seek psychotherapy they have a story to tell," psychologist Kenneth Gergen declared. Story making presumes interactive relationships. Historian Thomas Cole and behaviorist Bertram Cohler asserted that "neither lives nor texts can be understood apart from a complex interplay of participants," narrators, and listeners (Birren et al., 1996:131, 204, 61).

Taking into account criticisms concerning his model, Butler subsequently modified some points that he had emphasized in his 1963 article. In his 2002 contribution on "Life Review" for the *Encyclopedia of Aging*, for instance, Butler wrote:

> Life review is a progressive return to consciousness of memories and unresolved past conflicts for reevaluation and resolution. It is a normal, developmental task of the later years, a private process that differs with each individual. This evaluative process is believed to occur universally in all persons in the final years of their lives, although they may not be totally aware of it and may in part defend themselves against realizing its presence.
>
> (2002b:41)

Three key words—"progressive," "normal," and "developmental"—are as conspicuous in this 2002 definition as they had been in Butler's 1963 presentation. In both documents he underscored that life review could facilitate an individual's coming to terms with his or her past; yet he reissued his warning that clients could still end up with unresolved conflicts. And while encouraging younger persons to do life reviews, he continued to emphasize that older people's awareness of finitude generally prepared them for death in positive ways.

Rather than characterizing life review as a "universal process" (as he had done in 1963), Butler now accentuated the need for "evaluative" engagement with unconscious material (1963b). The argument he advanced in 2002 went beyond positing humans' innate capacity to retrieve past experiences to consciousness. Central now was his insistence that the process itself required intentionality. Coming to grips with one's own dying and death, he felt, justified a concerted effort to critique earlier situations that ground distinctive narratives into platforms for serious engagement with the inevitable.

FINAL REFLECTIONS ON LIFE REVIEW

A week before he died in 2010, Butler completed a draft of what proved to be his last restatement of life review. He intended "Prologue or Introduction to Life Review," reprinted in the appendix of this book, to preface a memoir he was writing primarily for his children. Butler also entertained the possibility that this text might preface a "brief book." Not only does his unexpected death make it worth analyzing, but the document affords us a chance to read how Robert Butler, then in his eighties, recapitulates aspects of his personal life and professional career.

There are nonetheless at least two risks in reading this document as a life review. First, while affirming that frailty affected the last years of his life, Butler gave no signs that he expected the end to come so soon. He had written about death in earlier life reviews; as we shall see, he elaborated on his thoughts in this "Prologue or Introduction" in words unmindful that he himself was at death's door. Second, there is no indication that he ever showed the document to anyone. There is a critical, dialogic element of life review missing in this text. Most life-review processes serve as a basis for remembering moments in situations shared between tellers and listeners, patients and clients. To be blunt, Butler's autobiographical passages here are not terribly self-revealing.

It is tempting to read more (and less) into Robert Butler's story than appears on the pages of this elusive text. Fortunately this document is only one of many statements from Butler, who declared that life reviews could take many forms. Accordingly, my reading of "Prologue or Introduction to Life Review" draws on Butler's insights about life review, the psychology of aging, and professional choices—observations made over his long career of writing, caring for patients, teaching, institution building, and devoting time to public service.

This manuscript incorporates previous writings. Butler includes here the same references to Aristotle, Bergman, and Maugham that originally appeared in his 1963 article. Significantly, Butler chose as a single epigraph William Cowper's quotation—"Mem'ry's pointing wand, that calls the past to our exact review"—which anticipated Butler's belief that memory work is valuable. The 2010 document abounds in references to other artistic and literary works, such as Montaigne, Jung, Camus's ruminations on suicide, Samuel Beckett's play *Krapp's Last Tape*, and John Bayley's tribute to his wife, *Elegy for Iris*. As before, science and literature complement each other in Butler's field of vision.

In the next pages of his final life review, rather than revisit childhood memories *de novo*, Butler decided to reprint verbatim "A Personal Note," the rendition of his early years published in *Why Survive? Being Old in America* (1975b:ix–x). Butler's account of his childhood remains as vivid in its detail and narrative line as it did when it first appeared thirty-five years earlier. Yet handling such rich material this way appears inconsistent with characterizing life review as an ongoing process that invites subjects to come to terms with painful, unresolved matters. Why did Butler choose not to interpret, with the advantage of late-life insights, the impact of his separation from his parents, poverty during the Great Depression, his grandfather's death, and his own life-threatening illness?

Perhaps the decision reflects his resilience and optimism: to his mind, his 1975 account sufficed in 2010. Writing for himself did not require an additional reflective lens. Other possibilities also exist. Perhaps he sensed that his early years fit Erik Erikson's model. Even if still traumatized by parental separation when he was eleven months old (when, according to Erikson, toddlers try to reconcile trust vs. mistrust) and his grandfather's death when Butler was seven (when Erikson claims that issues surrounding industry vs. inferiority are paramount), he may have determined that providing extra details might divert attention from central events of adulthood. After all, by any measure, he had succeeded beyond "mere survival." Perhaps he neither needed nor desired to stir up memories. The man who wrote pages later in "Prologue or Introduction" that "denial, in fact, is a very useful and natural, even necessary defense, an important psychological phenomenon," did not much like self-disclosure. Family, friends, and associates repeatedly note that he could be elliptical when talking about himself. In conversations I found him adept at deflecting issues and personalities that did not jibe with his sunny outlook on life. Butler could never name a single rival or enemy; instead he viscerally delighted in ways colleagues had enhanced his intellectual development and professional career.

Another interpretation is possible: Robert Butler knew how to be laconic while still disclosing something about himself. It is revealing, in my opinion, that Butler refers to himself as "I" more in this document than in any other piece of his published writing. And when I asked him to explicate his allusions to art critic Bernard Berenson, Leo Tolstoy's late diaries, and Mozart's sonatas—works he asked me to engage before our first interview— I sensed that they were, for him, codes for his encounters with God and divorce, subjects too difficult for him to articulate. Butler could be practical, as when advising elders "to travel to one's birthplace and attend reunions." Other asides—"More influenced by Martin Buber than Erik Erikson, I have been especially impressed by the moral dimension attending 'life reviews'"—remain tantalizingly suggestive. I cannot say whether they were the inner thoughts of an investigator recognizing limits to the scientism and positivism he extolled. Butler's appreciation of life review's "moral dimension" parallels what Rabbi Zalman Schachter-Shalomi called "life repair" in *From Age-ing to Sage-ing* (1995:116).

Opportunities and risks that Butler ascribed to late life amplify his views on adulthood:

> While the life review may emerge during many life crises, it is only at the end of life, in old age, that one has the opportunity to look back on the entire life course. Schopenhauer wrote that "A complete and adequate notion of life can never be attained by anyone who does not reach old age; for it is only the old man who sees life whole and knows its natural course; it is only he who is acquainted—and this is most important—not only with its entrance,

like the rest of mankind, but with its exit too; so that he alone has a full sense of its utter vanity; whilst others never cease to labor under the false notion that everything will come right in the end." . . .

We inch along in our fifties and sixties, even seventies and eighties, only beginning to question what we have done and re-evaluating relationships. As we grow still older and approach death, it becomes enormously important to strengthen our intimate relationships, to understand ourselves and our loved ones better, to come to grips with guilt and shame, experience remorse and serve others as well as effect reconciliations. We may come to confront and resolve acts of guilt by commission and omission through atonement and expiation. We may confess and seek forgiveness. Contrition may be sought. . . . The life review is not to be prettified. It is not peaches and cream. It must confront unresolved issues and dark negativism. It can result in a serious depression, especially if done without help.

(2010b)

This passage elaborates several themes Butler often expressed (without this much emphasis) in talking about aging amid the Longevity Revolution. "The life review is not to be prettified," he contends. Despite reservations and trepidations about the task, those approaching the end of their lives usually want to review their "natural" life course in the fullness of time. Did Butler follow his own prescription? The narrator reveals another critical turn in his process of self-inquiry.

How curious that Butler, an optimist, quotes approvingly from saturnine Arthur Schopenhauer (1788–1860). Ripening insight, claimed Schopenhauer, liberated "the man of mature age" from the whims, prejudices, and phantoms of boyhood and youth: "The chief result gained by experience of life is *clearness of result*. . . . it is only then that he sees things quite plain, and takes them for that which they really are" (Schopenhauer, [1890] 1970:134). This sentiment surely underscores the promising results of conducting a life review. Butler also shared Schopenhauer's conviction that judgment could ripen even as critical acumen waned. "Constantly finding new uses for his stores of knowledge and adding to them at every opportunity, he maintains uninterrupted that inward process of self-education which gives employment and satisfaction to the mind, and thus forms the due reward of all its efforts," declared Schopenhauer in "The Ages of Life" (79). "All this serves in some measure as a compensation for decreased intellectual power" (156–57). While not accepting Schopenhauer's presumption of diminishing intellectual capacities, nor his reliance on astrological signs to delineate the life course, Butler concurred that years brought ripening maturity to those who learned to make the most of their experiences.

Accordingly, Butler at the end of his life seems to adopt a different tone and emphasis in 2010 than in earlier renditions of life review. First, Butler, no churchgoer, intersperses theological terms (such as "atonement" and "expiation") among terms and phrases that clinicians and therapists are more accustomed to use. Second, he expands at length about negative patterns in attitudes and behavior that recur (perhaps even magnify) in relationships during old age. This leads him, third, to restate more forcefully than before his contention that life review does not simply entail a subject's indulging in "peaches and cream." Life review, like the human condition itself, requires disciplined introspection to pierce convenient half-truths. Getting past self-justification and offering reconciliation presuppose the honesty, resilience, and maturity to act in the here and now (Tavris & Aronson, 2007).

In this vein consider Butler's interpretation of recollecting past inadequacies in 1963 and 2010. In the first essay he observed that "the life review mechanism, as a possible response to the biological and psychological fact of death, may play a significant role in the psychology and psychopathology of the aged" (Neugarten, 1968:487). Younger people facing death or entangled in major crises often manifest the same signs of looking backward on life and looking forward to the end in a Janus-faced interrelationship. In his clinical judgment, Butler thought that most have grown receptive to overcoming their suspicions and reservations about life review. This is why many sought therapists' assistance in coming to terms with "the moment of truth" at the end of their lives.

Butler extends his reflections on death in the 2010 document—again, without any indication that he thought his own passing near. To him a "good death" occurs in the communal context of family and friends. This observation prompts two complementary lines of thought. On the one hand, while affirming that technology can "enhance hopes for a better death," he adds that a hospitalist might best serve as an *attending* physician" at bedside, and that nurses should defer to clergy and spiritual counselors. On the other hand, insofar as dying and death are fundamentally social acts, not just a matter of individual personhood, he suggests that facilitating suicide or "patient-controlled death" does not take account of the interests of bereaved family members and the community of survivors. Many ethical dimensions surrounding end of life, Butler recognized, remained unresolved.

Butler brackets reflections on death in his argument that older people must deal with their fears and traumas in the here and now. He extols "the therapeutic use of 'presentness'" (2010b:11–12), a phenomenon he compares to the "rediscovery of childhood." To envelop presentness demands internalizing a propensity to picture a life that unfolds in baby steps. Embracing this image opens elders to the possibility of enjoying the present moment in a childlike (not childish) manner. Closely associated with presentness in "an emotional vocabulary of pleasure," according to Butler, is "elementality," which evokes "the beneficence of nature." Over the life course people seize on the basics, he observes; from a fresh set of elemental priorities "emerges a layered accumulation of psychological, social, historical, and theological influences that reduces our relationship with nature" (17).

Hence Butler proposes ways to surmount fear in late life. Elders should try through life review to free themselves from being anxious because they are aware that time is running out. Older people ought to take delight in "the elemental things of life such as children, friendship, [and] human touching (physical and emotional)" (17). Invoking Bernard Berenson's descriptions of "life-enhancing experiences" that make "life a work of art," Butler envisions an old age that, for all its dark shadows, holds "still the opportunity for a sensuous appreciation of life" (19).

"Prologue or Introduction" demonstrated Butler's broadened field of vision about life review. The essay recasts both the value and cost of engagement in the therapy as it opens new vistas for integrating facets of the past that subjects might find useful later on. His final interpretation of life review concentrates on the here and now; it makes elementality critical to embracing one's self.

I read this piece as the mature reflection of someone who understood very well how to make fuller, richer use of life review as he advanced in years. Butler remained, to the end of his life, a scientist with a keen clinical eye and imaginative mind honed through critical thinking. In private Butler turned that therapeutic gaze on himself—deflecting issues at will. Well educated and remarkably urbane, he enjoyed collaborations with bright, congenial people in top-notch centers of learning and research. Butler always was receptive to fresh ideas; he wished to extract fundamental insights about human nature. He never compromised standards of excellence in his relentless search for truth. Indeed, it was his venturesome, playful curiosity set him apart from so many other talented gerontologists.

This 2010 document illuminates pathways to understanding the life course that Butler articulated in writings and speeches when he was well past the age that most of his peers retired. He was convinced that the Longevity Revolution, which added thirty years on average to human life in the United States over the past century, was altering the meanings and experiences of middle age and advancing years during the course of his lifetime. In "Prologue or Introduction" Butler moved beyond dualisms, which he had deployed over his career, juxtaposing positive features of advancing years (wisdom, healthfulness) with negative ones (decrepitude, frailty). He focused on the contributions elders could make to rising generations, defining legacy work as multidimensional. Not only does Butler value reminiscing as much as giving, but to him old age is a time in which people can shed inhibitions and conventions as they reveal their being. "Some evident characteristics of late life are markedly reinforced, such as the desire to leave a mark, by sponsoring and mentoring; by reminiscence and reflection, now more commonly welcomed, and *even by rebellion that follows the freedom from the need to earn one's daily bread*" (2010b:20). No doubt Butler, while composing that sentence, thought about how he might be remembered through his contributions to children, friends, and professional colleagues.

The call to rebellion had been implicit in Butler's writing all along, but only in later years did he attest to its importance to his life and career. It infused Butler's self-identification as a champion of the marginalized. Beneath his genuine affability and exquisite manners, Butler was a radical thinker, a rebel outraged by injustice, inequities, and ageism. Until recently I never fully appreciated the extent of the rage that informs *Why Survive?* I missed it, too, in his *A Generation at Risk: When the Boomers Reach Golden Pond* (1984). The subtitle refers to a 1981 film starring Katharine Hepburn, Jane Fonda, and Henry Fonda, but the text fans layers of disquiet concerning the nation's capacity to guarantee baby boomers a measure of social security comparable to what our parents and grandparents enjoyed. He also was raising the specter that the pond had been polluted as sources of freshwater ran out.

Feeling that he had so much more to do, Butler unflaggingly continued to write, speak, travel, advise, and espouse old-age causes. He encouraged younger people, especially baby boomers, to be pioneers in a global campaign to promote healthy aging as well as a salubrious environment. Butler was a "green" eminence grise.

For Butler, delving into life review meant grappling with potential opportunities and disadvantageous circumstances as an act of courage, itself a prelude to transformation. Engaging in life review, he knew from experience, gives elders license for moving on, ideally in a healthy manner. "Berenson spoke of 'making life a work of art,'" Butler recalled in his final life review. "This requires work, not wasting time on non-essentials and learning to say 'no.' It offers still the opportunity for a sensuous appreciation of life" (2010b:19). The completion of being was never finalized until the moment of death (Van Tassel, 1979). Still a work in progress, life's trajectories could be altered at will.

The process actually resembles a widening coil. The desire to revisit childhood, to return psychologically to earlier stages of life that were freed from anxiety and the restraints of time, observed Butler, enables older persons to liberate themselves from past commitments and constraints. Certain tasks of young adulthood and middle age, such as conquering fears of the unknown, remain imperative to the well-being of elders facing death.

Nonetheless, differences between youth and age matter. As Butler put it, "When a young person writes a novel he writes an autobiography; when an old person writes an autobiography he writes a novel" (12). Novels and autobiographies, both creative acts of self-expression, are neither easy to begin nor easy to complete. Not everyone is ready to delve into such modes of writing. Yet, paradoxically, few can afford to avoid the challenge. Sooner or later most older people, consciously or not, engage in the process of life review.

> Neither recalcitrant resignation nor exuberant self-satisfaction are the usual results of one's life review. There are many possible outcomes, not the least of which is the pleasure in survival itself in this tough, often confusing world. But review we should. . . . When in solitude there are many pitfalls. One does well to share one's life with others. It might just make possible a more helpful outcome.
>
> (BUTLER, 2010b)

In interviews with journalists and colleagues, he was candid—in a controlled way—about successes and disappointments over his career. A blogger interviewing Butler "was expecting an uplifting conversation about how we'll change aging with our vitality, health, and resourcefulness. That's not what I got." Butler pointed out that "we're not so healthy . . . also not so wealthy . . . we can't depend on our parents to pass along gobs of wealth to us. . . . [and] finally there are not enough caregivers to take care of us when we get ill and feeble." He reiterated his hope that boomers would be a transformative generation—even if they did not reap the benefits of their actions.

To the end of his life, Butler hewed optimistically to images of a good old age. Millions of women and men would benefit from the Longevity Revolution, he predicted. His persona and message gave audiences grounds for hope about prospects for their future selves.

To appreciate how Butler became the visionary of healthy aging, his life and contributions must be placed in historical context. Tracing his ways of thinking and implementing life review give us sense of what is to come. To

understand why he rose to be a giant in gerontology and geriatrics, however, requires us to trace how key moments and trends in postwar American history affected him and his contemporary researchers and practitioners in aging in postwar America. Butler changed as he matured, along
with institutions in which he trained, worked, and used to advance his
field. At the same time the nation underwent fundamental ideological, political, social, economic, and demographic shifts.

Butler's accomplishments and legacy were influenced by the pivotal
developments in postwar America. "We have come to see that the biographies of men and women, the kinds of individuals they have become, cannot be understood without reference to the historical structures in which
the milieu of their everyday life are organized," observed one of his teachers
at Columbia University, sociologist C. Wright Mills. "Historical transformations carry meanings not only for individual ways of life, but for the very
character—the limits and possibilities of the human being" (Mills, 1959:158).
A particular matrix of circumstances facilitated and frustrated Butler's efforts to change scientific minds and popular opinions about age and aging.
The political swing nationally from liberalism to conservatism over his adult
life thwarted his various attempts to enhance older people's well-being
through policy making.

Butler was no pawn, however. Given the varied circles in which he traveled, he had an uncanny sense of the contingent nature of the historical
times in which he lived. As he demonstrated in the 1963 essay on "The Life
Review," Butler willfully disregarded conventional wisdom. When proven
wrong, he quickly managed to cede positions and move on. Over time Robert Butler grew bolder in expressing critiques of the status quo that extended his customary age-based rhetoric; he took every opportunity to
enunciate recommendations for transformation on individual and societal
planes. In the process he sought to force major institutions to better serve
older people. That Butler did not wholly accomplish all that he intended
presents a challenge to those of us inspired by his legacy as we work in his
shadow.

two

THE FORMATIVE YEARS

Although in life reviews Butler downplayed the childhood trauma he experienced, he endured significant hardships growing up in the Great Depression. He suffered extended bouts of poverty, separation from parents, a grandfather's sudden passing, and his own brush with death. Yet there was enough love, happiness, and social support—provided by elders, teachers, a doctor, friends, and kindly strangers—to sustain the child's self-confidence in his ability to thrive, not merely survive. He went on to excel in high school. A stint in the Merchant Marines demonstrated his grit and leadership potential.

Hard knocks prepared Butler for the Ivy League. There, inspired teachers, challenging classmates, and editorship of Columbia's student newspaper groomed him to take intellectual risks, make connections, and respect the media. Medical school was less satisfying than undergraduate days, but here, too, instructors fed his curiosity and broadened his horizons. The newly minted physician was positioned to seize many advantages, professional and otherwise, offered in postwar America.

A CHILD OF THE GREAT DEPRESSION

The Great Depression had a greater impact on Butler's formative years, perhaps, than on others in his birth cohort. Hard times largely spared children of affluence, whereas those once broadly grouped together as "People of Plenty" (Potter, 1954) keenly felt the sudden reversal of resources. Widening scarcity after 1929 undercut middle-class Americans' sense of security. The Great Depression created havoc and caused despair for African Americans, single women, tenant farmers, day laborers, unskilled minorities, and displaced older workers. "Conditions varied across segments of the population, defined by age and sex, occupation, race, and residence," notes sociologist Glen Elder (1974:3). "Severe physical want and poverty were concentrated among the urban and rural lower classes."

Statistics attest to the severity of economic dislocation—the Depression cut deep and lasted a long time. But numbers alone do not convey the extent of psychic pain or widespread discontent (Kennedy, 1999; Lindenmeyer, 2005; McElvaine, 1993; McGovern, 2001). It is hard for subsequent generations to visualize faces etched with shame on people trying to maintain self-esteem; we barely hear their groans of misery (Gordon, 2009; McElvaine, 2008). Even we who endured a global recession, foreclosures, and budget crises only dimly sense what it must have been like. The current media chronicles taxpayers' anger and frustration; losses, fiscal and emotional, are widespread, here and abroad (Schwartz, 2011). Hitherto self-reliant, self-sufficient individuals have become dispirited, desperate, and doubtful that they will recover. That said, Butler and his peers spent childhood in conditions far worse than those we are facing today.

There exist surprisingly few reliable longitudinal studies focusing on the immediate and long-term impact of the Great Depression on the status and personality development of boys and girls born just before the stock market plummeted. In my opinion, Glen Elder's use of the Oakland Growth Study, originally collected in 1931, for *Children of the Great Depression* offers the best lens for reconstructing Robert Butler's childhood. Elder, who studied the physical, intellectual, and social development of 167 boys and girls born in 1920–21 through the 1930s, concluded that "the most striking

theme is the extraordinary degree of similarity, both academic and social, among youth with widely diverse backgrounds in the Depression"
(1974:138).

Born in New York City on January 21, 1927, Robert Neil Butler was the
only offspring of a broken marriage between David Frank Marcus and
Easter Carol Butler.° Butler described his early years in "A Personal Note"
introducing *Why Survive? Being Old in America*:

> My grandparents reared me from infancy. My parents separated shortly
> after my birth, and when I was eleven months old, my mother brought me to
> live with her parents in Vineland, New Jersey, where my grandfather, then in
> his seventies, was a gentleman chicken farmer. . . . He disappeared suddenly
> when I was seven. . . . I knew before they told me that he was dead. . . .
>
> It was my grandmother in the years that followed who showed me the
> strength and endurance of the elderly. This was during the Depression. We
> lost the farm. She and I were soon on relief, eating government-surplus food
> out of cans with stigmatizing white labels. Grandmother found work in a
> sewing room run by the WPA, and I sold newspapers and fixed bicycles for
> ten cents an hour. We moved into a hotel. When I was eleven, it burned to
> the ground with all our possessions. We started again. And what I remember
> even more than the hardships of those years was my grandmother's trium-
> phant spirit and determination. Experiencing at first hand an older person's
> struggle to survive, I was myself helped to survive as well.
>
> (1975b:IX–X)

°According to Social Security records, at the time he applied for a card (October 7,
1940), Robert Butler was still known as Robert Neil Marcus. According to the 1910
federal census, his mother (also known as Easter Carol Butter) was born in Oklahoma
around 1905; his father, who is listed in the same census, was born around 1896 and
lived on East 65th Street in Manhattan. As we shall see, Robert was raised in Vineland,
New Jersey, by his maternal grandparents. Fayette R. Dikeman (or Dilleman) was born
in Vermont circa 1856 and moved to Oklahoma before returning east. He married Ida,
who was born in New York in 1858. For Dikeman, see also http://www.archives.com/GA
.aspx?FirstName=Fayette+R&LastName=dikeman. I thank Wyneth Carter Achenbaum
and Janice Ryan for assistance in doing this genealogical research.

Loveless relationships, immature parenting, and financial exigencies caused many parents to abandon children in the 1920s and 1930s. So did abuse of spouse, elder, or child; alcoholism; physical, mental, or occupational disability; unemployment; and vagrancy or criminal activities. Children from broken homes customarily were entrusted to grandparents, since foster care and almshouses were grim alternatives.

Butler dealt with significant losses amid dire times. A serious bout with scarlet fever followed the departure of his septuagenarian "gentleman chicken farmer" without warning or explanation. In interviews and publications, however, Butler declared that he was made to feel special; he never expressed anger (though he alluded to shame) in recounting his Depression experiences. Friends and colleagues in eulogies noted Butler's ability to see good in virtually every setback.

As an adult Butler took pride in his ability to outlive early adversity. His indomitable grandmother regaled him with stories about Geronimo and reminisced about the outlaw Jesse James. Besides exposing the boy to classical music (which became a lifelong passion), she introduced him to books such as *Oliver Twist*. Hardship forced Butler to develop good judgment in youth, resourcefulness, and a discerning eye.

Much of Butler's early years, in fact, conform to developmental trends that Glen Elder illuminated in *Children of the Great Depression*. "To understand why some persons successfully adapt to challenging situations and others do not require knowledge of their resources and motivation, the support provided by the family and larger environment, and characteristics of the event or situation itself" (1974:12). Although the Depression certainly could have squelched his prospects for success, hard times did not extinguish Butler's sense that he was loved; by his account, he was nurtured to rise above hardship.

Butler knew by age seven that he wanted to be a doctor. The timing no doubt was influenced by fond memories of helping his grandfather "tend to the sick chickens." Dr. Rose, "our elderly, white-haired family physician," became another role model. In addition to explaining his grandfather's death, Dr. Rose saved his young life. Butler also admired Dr. Martin Arrowsmith, that fictional and younger version of Dr. Rose who was the hero of Sinclair Lewis's novel (1925). Although Butler briefly entertained other careers during his senior year of college, his resolve to become a doctor was quite steadfast. In a book published a few months before he died, he affirmed that he had rightly chosen a career that enabled him to advance best medical practices by rallying patients to healthful living:

> We can use our wisdom to identify what we desire in our lives: To improve ourselves, our lives, our health, our relationships, enhance our longevity, and to amend our lifestyle. . . . *The Longevity Prescription* seeks to engage you in a process by which your understanding of longevity science informs the way you live your life. Some of the best clinicians, scientists, physicians, and researchers in the world are focusing their energies on understanding aging, but your commitment to living long and well is required.
>
> (2010a:20–21)

Butler the medical researcher still manifested a child's desire to harness science's healing powers.

This youthful ability to envision a life richer than warranted by hard times fits Glen Elder's observation that "what young Americans in the 30s lacked was opportunity, not desire or ambition." Butler made the most of resources within his reach during the Great Depression. He adapted ways of thinking and behaving as appropriate. Besides his esteem for grandparents and Dr. Rose, Robert Butler enjoyed playmates who lived next door. Elementary school teachers pushed a bright but (admittedly) indifferent student to improve his grades. Emotional stress, postulated Elder, spurred "adaptive potential, in addition to resources and motivation" (Elder, 1974:293, 120, 37–38).

Like many *Children of the Great Depression,* Butler matured fast: "Economic hardship and jobs increased [his] desire to associate with adults, to 'grow up' and become an adult." He figured out survival techniques while watching his grandmother, other adults, and peers cope with adversity with steely determination. Butler learned to value "things that matter" in life (Elder, 1974:82, 282).

In 1941 Butler left Vineland for New York City when his mother remarried. There he passed entrance exams with high enough scores to attend DeWitt Clinton High School, a subway ride away from 91st Street in

Manhattan to a 21-acre campus in the Bronx. One of the great secondary schools in the nation, DeWitt Clinton catered to smart children of immigrants, preparing them for the nation's most rigorous colleges and professional schools. It was also the largest high school in the world during the 1930s, enrolling more than 12,000 boys (Jackson 1995:332). The writer James Baldwin graduated in 1942, the year before Butler; playwright Neil Simon, the year after.

While Vineland's schools had not prepared Robert Butler adequately for the competition and intellectual pressures at DeWitt Clinton, his stepfather, Fred Schlatter, demanded that homework be completed. Butler initially elected not to enroll in De Witt Clinton's honors track; he considered this model of academic meritocracy undemocratic. A visit to the principal's office (also attended by Schlatter) was enough to change his mind. And as one of the few students attending classes on Yom Kippur, Butler attracted the attention of his English teacher and other faculty.

Butler did well at DeWitt Clinton. He was tapped for Arista, a national honor society, and elected to a student-run judiciary board. He scored 100 percent in the New York State Regents' exam in Latin at a time in which few secondary schools taught classics; on this occasion his Latin teacher Mr. Solomon told Butler that he was "a scholar and a gentleman," a compliment that made a lasting impression. Good grades secured admission to Columbia University, but Butler left to do his patriotic part.

In 1943 Columbia was the world's largest producer of naval officers: it enrolled 2,500 midshipmen, 200 Coast Guard soldiers, 400 officers getting advanced training, and more than 700 in the Navy College Training Program—most of whom would see action before getting a degree ("Education," 1943). Nicholas McKnight, the Columbia dean in charge of the college's war plant, tried to secure Butler a position in the U.S. Navy. His protégé was rejected because of flat feet, a major disqualifier (Perrott, 1946). Butler was not alone; between 1941 and 1943 the Selective Service disqualified 30 percent of the five million men aged eighteen to thirty-seven examined. So he joined the United States Merchant Marine.

Butler was assigned to a Liberty ship, which transported cargo in the Atlantic, Mediterranean, Baltic, and Pacific oceans. Serving in the Merchant Marines was hazardous duty. One out of twenty-six mariners died in the line of duty during World War II—the highest percentage of fatalities for any military branch (Felknor, 1999). And because the ships were hastily and shoddily assembled, Liberty vessels often broke at the seams. (Some 1,500 instances of fractures were reported during World War II [Elphick, 2006].) Butler's vessel split on two separate occasions, requiring the adolescent to take charge temporarily. Leadership was thrust upon Butler several times over his two-year tour of duty; his superiors were too drunk or scared to take command.

Historical events in his formative years thus prepared Butler to handle vicissitudes in adulthood. This child of the Great Depression had overcome death and material losses. By age seventeen he had excelled in a high school for which he was ill prepared, seen much of the world in a leaky vessel, and learned leadership skills under fire. No wonder Butler was ready for whatever challenges Columbia University had to offer.

THE COLUMBIA UNDERGRADUATE YEARS

When he resumed coursework at Columbia after the war, Butler was immersed in the world of ideas in a privileged setting at a special moment in the history of U.S. higher education. Columbia was one of the nation's most prestigious universities at the beginning of the twentieth century—by some criteria, the best in the land. The Carnegie Foundation for the Advancement of Teaching in 1908 reported that Columbia surpassed Harvard, Johns Hopkins, Yale, Chicago, Michigan, Stanford, and Princeton in terms of endowment, instructional budgets, and scholarships (Cole, 2010:32–33). Columbia achieved elite status under two university presidents, scientist Frederick A. P. Barnard (who served from 1864 to 1889) and philosopher Nicholas Murray Butler (who served from 1901 to 1945). Both concentrated on building graduate programs offering highly specialized training. Columbia produced first-rate researchers and scholars as well as corporate executives and lawyers.

The cross-disciplinary course of studies that Butler pursued as a Columbia undergraduate had been refined over several decades by extraordinary pedagogues, roughly a third of the Faculty of Arts and Sciences, who deeply cared about training youth. The college, roughly the size of Amherst in the 1940s, incubated talent for the university's graduate and professional schools (McCaughey, 2003:287). Most graduates prospered in New York, though a Columbia degree served alumni well anywhere.

Initial inspiration for Columbia's liberal-arts curriculum came from John Dewey (1859–1952), a towering figure on the faculty from 1904 until 1930. "With respect then to both humanistic and naturalistic studies, education should take its departure from this close interdependence," Professor Dewey declared. "It should aim not at keeping science as a study of nature apart from literature as a record of human interests, but at cross-fertilizing both the natural sciences and the various human disciplines such as literature, economics, and politics" (1916:334). Dewey's pragmatic educational philosophy sought to inculcate ways of seeing and creating fresh possibilities within the existing order. "The aims and ideals that move us are generated through imagination. But they are not made out of imaginary stuff. They are made out of the hard stuff of the world of physical and social experience," he asserted in *A Common Faith* (Boydston, 1986:33). Building on Dewey's insight, Columbia College professors encouraged undergraduates to interact with peers and mentors. In due course, the faculty believed, students would learn how to conceptualize how puzzles came together.

Another architect of Columbia College's Core Curriculum was Pulitzer Prize–winning poet and critic Mark Van Doren, a faculty member from 1920 to 1959, who mentored such future luminaries as John Berryman, Whitaker Chambers, Allen Ginsburg, Thomas Merton, and Lionel Trilling. In *Liberal Education*, Van Doren expanded John Dewey's injunction to train minds for thinking critically, since "that makes the mind free to realize its choices." A traditionalist, Van Doren stressed basics in training minds: "All human work has its grammar, rhetoric, and logic; every man practices them his life long" (1959:129, 121, 83).

Jacques Barzun (1907–2012) also deeply affected the undergraduate community that Butler entered. Valedictorian of Columbia College's class of 1927 (the year Butler was born) and president of the Philolexian Society (a prestigious literary and debate club), Barzun taught at his alma mater from 1928 until his retirement in 1975. He was masterful in the classroom, regularly coteaching with literary critic Lionel Trilling a Great Books course in the Core. Butler remembered that class so fondly that Myrna Lewis later wanted to discover firsthand what sustained her husband's unbounded enthusiasm. Arrangements were made to permit her to audit the Great Books course in the early 1980s; the couple subsequently endowed the program with a $500,000 gift (Martineau, 2009).

For our purposes, Jacques Barzun's *Teacher in America* (published in 1947, when Butler was a Columbia undergraduate) deserves scrutiny for its impact on Butler's education. More like Dewey than Van Doren, Barzun felt that "education comes from within; it is a man's own doing, or rather it happens to him. . . . The sense of the plan can be seen at once by starting, not from the college, but from the world. What are the broad divisions of thought and action in the world? There are three and only three: we live in a world saturated with science, in a world beset by political and economic problems, in a world that mirrors life in literature, philosophy, religion, and the fine arts" (169). Columbia College, Barzun proudly proclaimed, was "highly representative of modern instruction through the country," thanks to its honors program, small interdisciplinary classes, flexible scheduling, innovative teaching modules and the "abandonment of loose electives" that encouraged premature specialization (168).

When Butler resumed undergraduate studies, the Columbia College Core Curriculum was undergoing modifications—part of an ongoing self-evaluation process as the United States became a superpower.

[The] three two-year sequences in science, the social sciences, and the humanities have brought us, we believe, to the point at which the younger student is offered a comprehensive view of what goes to the making of an intelligent citizen of the world. The salutary influence of these courses upon the mental consciousness and capacities of our students has been accepted by all but an almost negligible minority of the students themselves; and the merging of previously divided interests in the departments of our instruction, as well as the broadening effect of this merging upon the instructors who have conducted the courses, are probably results of no less importance to the well-being of college education.

(*A COLLEGE*, 1946)

The Columbia faculty sought to counterbalance their Eurocentric bias and to make the curriculum more amenable to cross-disciplinary inquiries.

Curricular reform was a priority elsewhere. A dozen Harvard professors, in consultation with hundreds of "persons of various walks of life and sections of the country," prepared *General Education in a Free Society*. The report, sometimes called *The Red Book*, presented "a view of the total American scene." It focused on character building, which instilled "initiative, zest, and interest, strength and driving power . . . regulated by the rules of fair play and a concern for the common good" (Buck et al., 1945:xiv, v, 262). Meanwhile the University of Chicago offered what Columbia sociologist Daniel Bell characterized as "the flavor of an aristocratic critique of the democratic—perhaps one should say populist— foundations of American education" (Bell, 1966:15; see also Beam, 2008; McNeill, 1991:36).

Columbia, Harvard, and Chicago, the major trailblazers of general education at midcentury, stoked the power of ideas to nurture consilience, civility, and character. Each sought "to free a student from provincialism and to lead him to self-discovery through an awareness of tradition, to confront him with the persistent issues of morals and politics, and to give him an understanding of the interconnectedness of knowledge" (Bell, 1966:50– 51). Preparing men to become leaders in major spheres of influence required something more than mastering elementary competencies or specialized knowledge. It presumed a liberal education that fostered creativity in a disciplined manner, at once mindful of the complementarities and discontinuities in human thought and behavior. It demanded receptiveness to fresh ideas in unfamiliar contexts. This was precisely the sort of education designed to instill confidence, intellectual and otherwise, in men like Butler and his peers.

These three universities faced logistical challenges after World War II, however, in reforming undergraduate education as they accommodated returning veterans. By September 1946 officials and students, facing enrollments in all of Columbia's units that topped 37,000 students, had to deal with makeshift housing and crowded classrooms. On the bright side, the surge in matriculation improved the university's budget sheet. In his last year of office (1944–45), President Nicholas Murray Butler turned a $1.6 million deficit into a $65,000 surplus (Cole, 2010:180; McCaughey, 2004).

More than at Harvard or Chicago, Columbia College's incoming students were children of immigrants, who represented roughly half of the undergraduate population. So when Professor John Erskine, an architect of the Core who taught at Columbia from 1909 to 1937, sought to foster "the basis for an intellectual life in common," he assumed that graduates would not go home again (McCaughey, 2003:297). "Whatever else the Columbia freshman may have felt after joining the College," the faculty hoped, "he could be in no doubt that he was exposed to an intellectual experience and was subject to demands qualitatively different from those of secondary school" (Bell, 1966:viii).

Students then and afterwards understood Erskine's position. Thus Norman Podheretz, who graduated from the college in 1948 (a year before Butler), called the experience of leaving Brownsville for Morningside Heights "a brutal bargain," but one he willingly made (McCaughey, 2003:297). Stephen J. Trachtenberg '59, who served as president of George Washington University for nearly two decades, extolled the Core's "transformational effect on my world view. It defined what it meant to be an educated person, and the courses I took, the books I read, and the people—professors and classmates—have informed my personal and professional life" (Meyer, 2010).

Like Podheretz and Trachtenberg, Butler felt that Columbia nurtured in him an intellectual cast of mind that stimulated his later success. He credited "this Core Curriculum with teaching him to think broadly across subjects, a skill that was vital to his research" (Martineau, 2009). Teachers there, in his opinion, considered grappling with ideas a serious vocation. Butler took full advantage of Columbia's educational resources.

Unlike most undergraduates then and now, Butler made a point of getting to know professors. He often visited the office of John Herman Randall Jr. (1899–1980) who, after earning his degrees at Columbia, taught philosophy and cultural history on the faculty from 1921 to 1967. Butler proudly showed me his copy of Randall's *Making of the Modern Mind* (1926), a textbook commissioned for the Core. Butler got to know well French scholar Donald Murdoch Frame, a navy veteran and assistant to the dean of the college from 1946 to 1950. He interacted with Howard Levi, who wrote a text for the Core on mathematical problems and procedures, and political scientist Joseph Perkins Chamberlain, who was fond of quoting Walt Whitman's aphorism "And nothing endures but personal qualities." Such initiatives reveal something about how Butler's curiosity and affability stimulated intellectual breadth.

One of Butler's favorite instructors was Ernest Nagel (1901–85), a logical positivist who integrated John Dewey's instrumentalism into philosophy and the sciences. (Particularly appealing was Nagel's seminar, taught with Paul Lazarsfeld, on social-science methodology.) Butler took to heart Nagel's insistence that facts should bury ill-conceived ideas (Suppes, 1994). The lesson took hold: Butler throughout his career embedded speeches and writings with hard evidence that buttressed possibilities for improving the quality of late life.

That Butler took many science courses at Columbia College underscores the importance of the field in postwar America. In *Endless Horizons*, Vannevar Bush, the nation's top scientific administrator in World War II, flatly declared, "Without scientific progress no amount of achievement in other directions can insure our health, prosperity, and security as a nation in the world" (1946:42). According to Harvard's *Red Book*, science provided "the material basis of the good life" and "directly fostered the spiritual values of humanism" (Buck et al., 1945:50).

Science education at Columbia, by general account, did not have the standing it enjoyed at other schools. Size was a factor: with relatively fewer undergraduates to teach, the college and university did not have as many scientists on the faculty or key administrative posts as MIT, Stanford, Johns Hopkins, Michigan, Cornell, or Harvard. During Butler's undergraduate years, science was running "on momentum rather than new fuel" (Cole, 2010:131; McCaughey, 2003:398–401).

Still, Butler had access to distinguished scientists at various stages of their careers. William von Eggers Doering, an assistant professor of chemistry, did research on quinine while establishing on campus the Hickrill Chemical Research Foundation to underwrite postdoctoral research (Doering, 1990–91). Butler also worked with microbial geneticist Francis J. Ryan (1916–63), whose courses on vertebrate zoology showcased his love of science and passion for teaching. "Professor Ryan took a callow underclassmen from Washington Heights, brash and argumentative as precocious students often are, and turned me into a scientist," Nobel laureate Joshua Lederberg recalled. "He took me seriously enough to discipline my thinking, which was exactly what I needed right then" (Lederberg, n.d.).

Charles R. Dawson, who taught more than 100,000 Columbia undergraduates organic chemistry from 1939 until his retirement in 1979, was Robert Butler's adviser. (Dawson's son recalled that his father reworked lecture notes every time he taught.) In addition, Dawson wrote 120 scientific papers on the biochemistry of plants. As assistant dean of Columbia College (1944–55), he oversaw the premedical program. Butler credits his mentor with helping him gain entrance into Columbia University's medical school, the College of Physicians and Surgeons. Undoubtedly, extracurricular contributions also increased Butler's chances for admission.

Undergraduate life, even at heady places like Columbia, did not revolve solely around classes. Butler told me that he enjoyed exploring New York City. He frequented museums and walked to Harlem to hear jazz. Students tended to learn a lot in the company of peers, especially since there were strictures about too much fraternizing with faculty. "Let me say bluntly, as I do not hesitate to do when my students broach the subject, that friendship between an instructor and a student is impossible," Jacques Barzun declaimed. "This does not mean that the two should remain strangers; there can exist cordial, easy relations, tinged perhaps with a certain kind of affection; but friendship, not. For friendship has strict prerequisites, among them, freedom of choice and equality of status" (Barzun, 1947:222).

Respectful of boundaries, Butler sought to model his faculty mentors. Barzun appeared on the cover of *Time* because he was a public intellectual as well as a master teacher. Likewise, Butler indicated to me that working for the *Columbia Daily Spectator* was a vehicle for his voice to be heard beyond the classroom. Peer support was critical. When Butler went to work for the college newspaper, several close friends joined him on the staff. Paul Mishkin, who became a distinguished law professor, nominated him to be editor-in-chief. Another classmate, Vincent Carrozza, later a successful businessman and Columbia trustee, served as the business manager. A third friend, Reed Harris, would later help Butler edit *Human Aging*, a major National Institute of Mental Health study, in the 1960s.

Founded in 1877, the *Columbia Daily Spectator* was, after the *Harvard Crimson*, the second longest continuously operating college news daily in the United States. Butler fielded three big stories: the selection of Dwight D. Eisenhower as president of Columbia (he made editorial decisions to break a few rules by publishing a special commemorative issue); the publication of Alfred Kinsey's report on *Sexual Behavior in the Human Male*, for which he interviewed Ruth Benedict; and an investigation into faculty politics after the publication of the latest report on the Core Curriculum. Writing three hundred editorials under deadline honed Butler's prose. Besides learning "how to boss people around," as he put it to me, Butler came to appreciate how journalists framed controversial ideas while cultivating and maintaining media contacts in order to interview subjects more accomplished in age and experience. He tapped these skills throughout his career.

Butler was initiated into the Philolexian Society of Columbia in 1949, the year he graduated. Founded in 1802, Philo is the oldest organization on campus. Members included essayist Randolph Bourne; poets Joyce Kilmer, John Berryman, Richard Howard, and John Hollander; publishers Robert Giroux and Jason Epstein; Trappist monk Thomas Merton; a New York Giants quarterback; two mayors of New York, a Supreme Court justice, members of Congress, and ambassadors. Although not elected to Phi Beta Kappa (because of a poor grade in German), Butler demonstrably possessed the necessary brains and energy for Columbia's College of Physicians and Surgeons.

MEDICAL TRAINING

Columbia was the first institution in the British colonies to confer medical degrees (1767), though the medical department, the College of Physicians and Surgeons, was not fully integrated into the university until 1891. The College of Physicians and Surgeons became coeducational in 1917. The faculty established what became the Mailman School of Public Health a year later to teach public-health principles to medical students (McCaughey, 2003:171; Rosenfield, 1998:201–2). Throughout the nineteenth century, the college trained men to practice medicine in their local communities. The relationship between physicians and hospitals was "a marriage of convenience" (Rosenberg, 1987). Tuition and patient fees rarely covered expenses. The federal government after the Civil War supported agricultural science but left financing medical research to universities (Dupree, 1986).

The College of Physicians and Surgeons received mixed reviews in Abraham Flexner's *Medical Education in the United States and Canada*. Flexner praised the school's laboratories, citing the anatomy lab as one of "the most elaborate plant of its kind." But he deplored its lack of a library and small endowment. Claiming that New York's medical institutions could make it the "Berlin or Vienna of the continent," he leveled the criticism that Columbia's clinical facilities impeded "effective scientific or pedagogic use . . . for laboratory and clinical teaching" (1910:268, 275). To improve its standing, the College of Physicians and Surgeons needed to follow Johns Hopkins's model, which, after 1893, placed medical students in hospital wards to work under their professors' direction.

President Nicholas Murray Butler must have anticipated Flexner's recommendation that the College of Physicians and Surgeons create a scientific medical facility and affiliate with a teaching hospital: in 1910, he announced plans to build a new medical center in conjunction with Presbyterian Hospital, using a $2 million gift from the Vanderbilts. After more than a decade of bickering over site and finances, the Columbia-Presbyterian Medical Center opened in 1928 (McCaughey, 2003:305–8).

"The primary place for medical research is in the medical schools and universities," observed Vannevar Bush (1946:52–53), noting that between the world wars the United States had assumed world leadership in this area. "It is clear that if we are to maintain the progress in medicine which has marked the last 25 years, the Government should extend financial support to basic medical research in the medical schools and in the universities, through grants both for research and for fellowships." There were modest increases in federal allocations for medical research after World War I; the great infusion in grants and fellowships would not come until the mid-1950s. A prime beneficiary of new dollars, the College of Physicians and Surgeons became a major revenue source for the university (Bell, 1966:295; Dupree, 1986:331–32).

Butler thus entered a medical school in transition, a place where research was to bridge the aims of advancing science and healing patients. Impediments remained. Congress rejected proposals in 1949 and 1951 to extend federal grants for institutional grants and medical-student loans and scholarships (Strickland, 1972:250–51). Some worried, moreover, that too much emphasis was being placed on specialization in professional schools: "Men are not narrow in their intellectual interests by nature," observed Princeton economics professor Jacob Viner in 1950. "It takes special and rigorous training to accomplish that end" (Viner, 1950).

In at least four respects, however, students who had strong liberal-arts backgrounds mitigated Viner's concerns. The educational environment permeating the College of Physicians and Surgeons resembled the milieu that Butler had experienced at Columbia College: First, most of the faculty were dedicated instructors as well as gifted investigators. The best teachers enjoyed great prestige for their scientific work, and vice versa. Second, whatever their area of specialization, most of the professors that Butler encountered at the College of Physicians and Surgeons crossed scientific boundaries in the pursuit of knowledge. Third, competition for admission into the first-year class was intense. Fourth, as was the case in his undergraduate years, intellectual engagement with classmates was an important part of Butler's educational formation.

In the 1950s getting into medical school required advanced planning and very good grades. According to a survey of the medical class of 1957, 44 percent of those matriculating knew where they were headed at least four years before entering the College of Physicians and Surgeons. At least half reported "a great deal of competition" as undergraduates (Thielens, 1958). There was room for vacillation. As a senior Butler toyed with becoming an entrepreneur with his friend Henry O'Neill, whose grandparents owned Peru's leading newspaper. To cover his bets while he settled on a career, he fulfilled all of his pre-med requirements.

The day that Butler took examinations to enter medical school, he decided at the last minute to go to a formal. He called his good friend (and president of the class of 1949) Robert Milch to fix him up with a date. Milch introduced Butler to a very attractive woman, Diane McLaughlin, a one-time Barnard student who (among other things) shared his taste for Pall Mall cigarettes. The pair, hitting it off, decided to marry in 1950, after Butler's graduation from college. The couple lived in Fort Lee, New Jersey, across the river from Columbia; Diane worked in the dean's office of the College of Physicians and Surgeons while Butler was in medical school. The Butlers' first child, Chris, was born in 1951; their second, Carole, was born three years later, during his internship.

As he had done in the college, Robert Butler worked closely in medical school with an extraordinary company of researchers-clinicians-professors. He got to know the dean, Willard Cole Rappeley, MD—whom Nicholas Murray Butler characterized as a "corker" and Jacques Barzun described as a "baron." While Dr. Rappeley was at the helm (1931–58), teaching and research budgets of the College of Physicians and Surgeons increased sixfold and twenty-five-fold, respectively. A friend of Fiorello LaGuardia's and a man respected by peers for "erudition and action," Dean Rappeley somehow found time to head the Josiah Macy Jr. Foundation (1941–65), then and now one of the nation's most creative centers underwriting cross-disciplinary medical education and research (Bowers, 1978:879–80).

Butler also learned techniques for understanding diseases and bodily functions from some of the most eminent medical scientists of the day. For instance, he worked with Dr. Dickinson Woodruff Richards Jr. (1895–1973), who won a Nobel Prize for developing cardiac catheterization and drugs effective in alleviating several heart diseases (Cournard, 1989). In Hans Thacher Clarke, who used his association with Kodak and support from the Chemical Foundation to build a strong faculty and top-flight laboratories in biological chemistry, Butler saw a distinguished experimental researcher train doctoral candidates and medical students beyond the basics of organic chemistry and biology (Vickery, 1975).

Given the important collaborative roles that women scientists and gerontologists played later in Butler's career, it merits mention that he studied under some distinguished female professors and researchers at the College of Physicians and Surgeons. Dr. Virginia Apgar (1909–74) trained in anesthesia after being discouraged from pursuing surgery. The first woman to become a full professor in the medical school, Apgar virtually created the field of neonatology (Pearce, 2005). Apgar tests are still used to evaluate the health of newborns. Virginia Kneeland Frantz, MD, the first woman surgical intern at Presbyterian Hospital, was a member of the faculty from 1924 to 1962. Frantz "challenged her students to replace rote memory with constructive and critical thought" (Christy, 1995). Butler also worked with Margaret Murray, MD, who served forty years on the faculty. In collaboration with surgeon and pathologist Arthur Purdy Stout, Murray focused her research on cellular neurobiology; in later years she was a visiting scientist at the National Institutes of Health (Bornstein, 1989).

Butler respected pediatrician Rustin McIntosh, who drew the best out of students in clinical experiences on hospital wards (Damrosch, 1966). He admired Calvin H. Plimpton, MD, later president of Amherst College, the Downstate Medical Center (Brooklyn), and the American University of Beirut. Butler asked clinical professor Kermit L. Pines to take care of his mother and stepfather in their later years (Palladino, 2010).

Like many of his classmates, Butler had mixed opinions about Robert Frederick Loeb (1895–1973), coauthor of a classic textbook, who became chair of the Department of Medicine in 1947. Feelings ranged from awe over his erudition (an honors graduate of the University of Chicago, Loeb nearly quit medical school before ending up first in his class at Harvard) to fear over having to bear the brunt of one of his cutting remarks—though Loeb claimed to have loved all his students. Loeb, an internist, believed that in "undergraduate medical education we maintain the emphasis on intellectual growth, and that we guard against the dilution of our efforts"

(1963:579). He urged students to imagine what they would want done to them if they were patients confined in a hospital bed.

Medical school in itself did not spark Butler's interest in senescence. He knew that Loeb had done work in the area of geriatrics, but this was not an interest they shared. Butler also worked with Henry Simms, MD, a clinician studying cellular aging and charter member (1945) of the Gerontological Society, and had read about Clive McCay's research into the effect of caloric reduction on the life expectancy of rats (Strickland, 1972:38). While aging was not then part of the medical-school curriculum, Columbia encouraged medical students to pursue their own scientific curiosity and research interests. To this end, the College of Physicians and Surgeons armed them with good techniques and taught them how to reason scientifically.

Medical school was a less supportive environment than college. Butler found dissecting a cadaver dehumanizing. Laboratory investigations seemed tedious and lonely. He got little empathy or positive feedback when he lost his first patient. Gallows humor did not comfort him. Butler told me that he chafed in a clinical research environment that put greater emphasis on results than relationships, a setting suffused with advice that William Osler (the foremost medical educator a half century earlier) gave to medical students—"Cultivate, then, gentlemen, such a judicious measure of obtuseness as will enable you to meet the exigencies of practice with firmness and courage, without, at the same time, hardening 'the human heart by which we live'" (Osler, 1889). Osler's bloodless equanimity made him uncomfortable. Here, then, may lie the origins of a trait that would characterize Butler's attitude toward colleagues who reified professional norms: he conformed to scientific rules and norms for advancing knowledge and caring for others, but he railed against practices that diminished dignity in patients and their caregivers that he was helping.

Butler claimed to have enjoyed greatly his internship (1953–54) in at the St. Luke's-Roosevelt Hospital Center, where he honed diagnostic skills and considered going into partnership with an internist. He disliked the long hours on the floors, sleepless nights, and quality of care he often gave when exhausted and poorly supervised. In addition to new friends, Butler deepened bonds with Jerold M. Lowenstein, a college buddy with whom he teamed up at the College of Physicians and Surgeons. With their wives, the pair took a road trip in 1952 in part to test Dr. Loeb's hypothesis that the best U.S. medical schools were located between Cambridge and Baltimore. After seeing Stanford, Chicago, and Washington University, the pair concluded that the "great" doctor just might have been wrong in some of his opinions.

Butler became interested in the problems of aging during his internship at St. Luke's. He enjoyed talking with elderly people. He wanted to know how they thought and felt about things. He was offended, moreover, by the disparaging terms that doctors and nurses used to describe older patients, such as "crock" and "GOMER—Get Out of My Emergency Room." So, deciding against a residency in internal medicine and hematology, he opted for psychiatry.

> In 1953, it began to hit me: a lot of patients I was seeing clearly had psychological, behavioral, and social issues, not just medical ones. It also occurred to me that we didn't know anything about aging. So both of these ideas were in my mind while I was training. . . . So that led me to pore through the books, and I found that some descriptions of older people with brain damage who actually became more agitated by the drug [Seconal] instead of less—a paradoxical drug reaction. I concluded that either I was asleep in class at Columbia or they never gave that lecture. So I thought, there is something about old age that I've got to know.
>
> (NORMAN, 1997)

Hence Columbia's value in shaping minds. Robert Butler became "the man who saw old anew," as a feature story in the *New York Times* would describe him decades later (Norman, 1997). Intrigued by a complex problem beyond his expertise, he did more than just read books on aging. Relying on positive experiences with grandparents and at the same time repulsed by the demeanor of health-care professionals in hospital wards, Butler sought to ascertain the big picture, guided by his own sense of how to proceed.

At this critical juncture, Butler trusted his instincts. Rather than complete the next phase of his professional education by following his Ivy

League peers to East Coast establishments, he chose to go across the country to a center where professionals were experimenting with a variety of approaches to mental-health issues afflicting older adults. A young man with a wife and two young children probably would not have taken such a risk were he not prepared to stretch. Confident of the skills, professional and personal, at his disposal, Butler was eager to pierce the veil of ignorance that impeded efforts by physicians and the public to understand the basics of aging.

three

A PROFESSIONAL APPRENTICE

Butler's decision to become a gero-psychiatrist was an unusual career path in the 1950s. Most psychiatrists treated children, adolescents, and young adults; mental illnesses afflicting the aged attracted little interest. Concurrently, psychiatry was undergoing a paradigm shift in America after World War II. Medical schools were revamping core curriculums and modifying residency requirements to take account of the explosion of knowledge in post-Freudian theories, specialists' appreciation of the neurobiology of psychiatric illness, and the advent of alternative methods of treatment (Haak & Kaye, 2009). The federal government's increasing interest and investment in research and training in the mental-health arena opened career paths unimagined a decade earlier.

Butler had to become board-certified to practice psychiatry, but as the field redefined its raison d'être, he encountered gatekeepers willing and able to accommodate his passion for understanding and caring for older adults. Far from being dismissed as an eccentric, the young physician found his professional niche while acquiring training that would serve him as a researcher and a clinician. His Columbia years undoubtedly prepared him for such intellectual risk-taking. Few other Ivy League peers would have chosen to affiliate with an unorthodox psychiatric institute on the West Coast. That experience, however, positioned him to join one of only two interdisciplinary teams of researchers in the United States that were investigating patterns of health and illness among older people.

To characterize Robert Butler as a "professional apprentice" is to underline anomalies in his status between 1954 and 1963. His apprenticeship did not proceed through a series of psychodynamic traineeships that culminated in establishing a private practice, as most psychiatrists did. Nor did he undergo psychotherapy at the beginning of his residency. Instead, he learned a lot about psychopharmacology. He worked with experts in disparate disciplines who shared his curiosity about late-life moods and behaviors. Because he proved a capable trailblazer, his mentors and senior investigators treated him like a colleague, not an acolyte. In these years Butler came into his own, professionally and otherwise.

LANGLEY PORTER INSTITUTE AT THE VANGUARD OF PSYCHIATRY'S PARADIGM SHIFT

The Langley Porter (Neuro)Psychiatric Institute in San Francisco opened in 1943 with great expectations. Its founders wanted to fight mental illness through research, training, and prevention. Building on the expertise available at the nearby medical school, they intended to capitalize on the clinical experiences gained through treating twenty-nine thousand patients in nine state hospitals. During the Great Depression, Langley Porter, MD, a professor of pediatrics and medical dean at the University of California, San Francisco (UCSF), lobbied with officials at the California Department of Mental Hygiene and with the president of the University of California system for a research center focusing on mental health. History was on Porter's side: he cited legislation proposed in 1913 that justified establishing a psychiatric hospital in the Bay Area (Ruesch, 1978; Statdman, 1967; University, 2010). Shortly after Dean Porter's retirement at age seventy in 1940, Karl Bowman, MD, was named director of the institute and first chair of the UCSF medical school's newly created Division of Psychiatry. He served as president of the American Psychiatric Association in 1946 ("Karl," 1973).

The new institute did not build on Sigmund Freud's psychoanalytic techniques and theories about human (sub)consciousness, which dominated mental-health professional practices and saturated popular culture in the United States throughout the 1940s (Brown, 1940; Burger, 2008). New developments in medical thinking and research, as well as discoveries in pharmacology and other basic sciences, spurred Bowman and his colleagues to consider alternative approaches to treating and dealing with mental illness in postwar America. Different, differential diagnoses of mental disorders challenged the neurological and psychiatric foundations of Freudian concepts. The Group for the Advancement of Psychiatry, founded in 1946 by William C. Menninger, mobilized "young Turks" to move their field beyond the traditional, institutional approaches advocated by the American Psychiatric Association (Menninger, 1948; Richardson, 1989). Meanwhile a growing number of psychiatrists and laypersons began to question whether there were fixed boundaries between "illness" and "normalcy" (Simon, 1948; Szasz, 1961).

For instance, the search for alternatives to existing paradigms prompted investigators to scrutinize the etiologies of disorders such as dementia paralytica, which afflicted roughly half the residents in psychiatric institutions. Once clinicians and researchers realized that the mania, grandiosity, and paralysis hitherto ascribed to dementia paralytica actually were manifestations of late-stage syphilis, they started to treat the causes, not the effects of the disorder (Nuland, 2003:176–81). Such breakthroughs justified experiments in psychiatry that brought biological approaches to bear on other affective maladies and major illnesses such as schizophrenia. Here, too, serendipity sometimes played a role in the process of scientific discovery. To wit: lithium was proven in 1949 to relieve the symptoms and to dampen the likelihood of extreme behavior in many cases of manic-depression—though no one at the time really knew why. (The etiology of bipolar illness, it is worth noting, is still unknown today.) Scientists after

World War II increasingly sought to infer the physiological course of this and other diseases by studying the "mechanisms of action" of pharmacological agents (Barondes, 1990; Gruenberg, 1977; Minnesota, 2010).

Amid discontent in professional circles and paradigmatic shifts in psychiatric theories of disease and therapeutic interventions, the federal government after World War II assumed leadership in the fight against mental illness. The National Mental Health Act (1946) authorized the establishment three years later of the National Institute of Mental Health (NIMH), one of the first four such centers on the Bethesda, Maryland, campus of the National Institutes of Health. Several circumstances gave greater national visibility to the problem of mental disorders, which historically had been the purview of state institutions and private individuals. According to James A. Shannon, MD, who directed the National Institutes of Health from 1955 to 1968, the enactment of the Social Security Act (1935) paved the way for federal lawmakers to actualize the "general welfare" phrase in the Constitution's preamble to benefit vulnerable citizens. It justified Washington's involvement in mental-health investigations (as it sanctioned research investments in cancer and public health generally). The National Institutes of Health, in concert with the National Science Foundation, had a mandate to prioritize intellectual and educational initiatives that advanced medicine and science for the national good. Partnerships with universities and other entities in the nonfederal research community produced breakthroughs in basic science. Fierce competition for prestige and profits sparked panacean dreams of discovering technological magic bullets and wonder drugs for cursed scourges (Brandt, 1987).

Other factors contributed. Over the decades, state institutions (like almshouses) had basically devolved into custodial sites, warehouses for men and women stigmatized by their disorders. Health-service professionals' experiences with the Selective Service and in combat zones during World War II, however, raised the possibility for developing alternatives to institutionalized nihilism. Psychodynamic psychiatry had proven beneficial to those who suffered from mental illness. By the 1960s a new generation of psychiatric leaders would be trumpeting policies that promoted deinstitutionalization and, less radically, designed rehabilitative strategies to enhance the quality of lives of those residing in facilities or dwelling in community-based settings (Grob, 1987; Shannon, 1967).

Changing perceptions within the scientific community and legislative bodies increased resources for people who were mentally ill. (A segment of the population that had been largely ignored or abandoned throughout U.S. history, mentally ill patients in many cases continue to grow old in dismal institutions.) Public allocations increased more than sixfold between 1940 and 1955, by which time federal dollars accounted for half the nation's spending on research and development. Nongovernmental research scientists in universities and at institutes such as Langley Porter became successful applicants in peer-reviewed competitions for research funds. This infusion of dollars expanded the scope of mental-health services in the United States. Nonfederal support increased twentyfold between 1948 and 1960. Whereas half the states in 1948 supported only institutional care, every state had mental-health programs by 1960 (Berliner & Kennedy, 1970). A variety of circumstances, in short, made it likely from the outset that Langley Porter would be a successful venture. The intellectual climate fostered innovations in dealing with mental illness.

PSYCHOPHARMACOLOGY AT LANGLEY PORTER

Seeking treatments complementary to psychotherapy after World War II, Dr. Karl Bowman and his principal co-investigator, Dr. Alexander Simon (a College of Physicians and Surgeons graduate), took intellectual gambles at Langley Porter. Administering an electric current through the brains of fifty-three patients with schizophrenia and bipolar (manic-depressive) illness, Bowman and Simon reported some improvement. They nonetheless concluded that the therapy was not beneficial in cases of psychoneurosis; it proved a more dangerous treatment, less easily administered, than electroshock (Bowman, 1939; Bowman & Simon, 1948). With colleagues from UCSF's divisions of psychiatry and neurosurgery, the Langley Porter research team offered "a controlled evaluation" of thirty-three psychotic patients six months after undergoing unilateral or bilateral lobotomies to treat their mental illness (Simon et al., 1951).

In the late 1940s Bowman and Simon launched research into the origins, behavioral characteristics, and treatment of problem drinkers, especially older alcoholics. Of particular note was the group's pharmacological approach to alcohol abuse. Joining with colleagues in UCSF's divisions of pharmacology and psychiatry, Bowman and Simon proposed that Antabuse had therapeutic value. This line of research continued for a decade, highlighting the high incidence of alcoholism among older subjects (Bowman et al., 1951; Hine et al., 1952; Macklin, Simon, & Crook, 1953; Simon, 1948).

As they fostered connections with researchers across UCSF's medical campus, Bowman and Simon recruited outsiders who would enrich multidisciplinary ways of thinking. Before Butler joined Langley Porter, Gregory Bateson served as a research associate in psychiatry and communications; he later accepted an appointment in Stanford University's anthropology department. Bateson's interest in alcoholism led him to work with UCSF psychiatrist Jurgen Ruesch, with whom he coauthored *Communication: The Social Matrix of Psychiatry* (1951) (Anton-Luca, 1998). Barely overlapping Butler's residency was social psychologist Marjorie Fiske (Lowenthal), who had honed her talent for interdisciplinary research at Columbia's Bureau of Applied Social Research, where she collaborated with Paul Lazarsfeld, Robert Merton, and C. Wright Mills. Professor Lowenthal's first major UCSF report, *Lives in Distress: The Paths of the Elderly to the Psychiatric Ward*, was based on 530 older people in psychiatric wards of San Francisco General Hospital. Through her grants and collaborations— along with Simon's work on the impact of deinstitutionalization and community mental initiatives on older people—Fiske helped establish Langley Porter as a major center for studying the social-psychological context of adult personality development and aging (Cahan & Yeager, 1967; Christ, 1961; Ernst et al., 1956; Fiske, 1960; Lowenthal, 1964a, 1964b; Simon, 1971, 1984).

Butler was intrigued by the work being done at the Langley Porter Psychiatric Institute; his interview with Alexander Simon concerning a possible residency there went well. He liked UCSF's clinical approach, which (unlike Columbia) put greater emphasis on the diagnostic recognition of syndromes than on basic science. The institute was small: its clinic annually took on five to six trainees supervised by a cadre of cross-disciplinary mental-health experts and psychologists in private practice who devoted several hours a week to training. Hence Butler saw his residency in San Francisco as an opportunity to learn about aging and mental health with instructors like Bowman and Simon (as well as Langley Porter associates such as Lester Margolis, MD), who were his early mentors (Katzman & Bick, 2000).

Butler joined the team at Langley Porter that was studying pharmacotherapy in psychiatry. He worked on chlorpromazine hydrochloride, an antipsychotic originally found useful by a French surgeon in calming patients recovering from anesthesia. Synthesized in 1950 and approved by the U.S. Food and Drug Administration four years later (after efficacious tests on some of the most hopeless cases in state institutions), chlorpromazine, according to French and U.S. researchers at the time, affected a variety of receptors in the central nervous system. The compound caused "sedation without narcosis"—hence its effectiveness in addressing various mental disorders, such as mania and psychomotor excitement. Chlorpromazine also offered a treatment for vomiting, and in some patients there was noticeable improvement in cognitive and emotional behavior.

As a treatment for schizophrenia, chlorpromazine quickly replaced electroconvulsive shocks and psychosurgery (Brunton et al., 2006; Healy, 2004). There were side effects, however, which ranged from weight gain and changes in skin pigmentation to possible anomalies in the reproductive system. "Although chlorpromazine and reserpine have been depicted as highly effective therapeutic agents by a legion of investigators, considerable disagreement still exists as to the value of these drugs," observed Langley Porter's Lester Margolis, a neurologist. "They have been described by some as worthless. . . . They have been described as both a valuable adjunct and as a hindrance to psychotherapy" (Margolis, 1957:698). Through the generation and dissemination of objective, evidence-based analyses, the institute's leadership hoped to create a niche for Langley Porter in psychopharmacology, an area that executives in major drug companies were finding to be a lucrative market (American Medical Association [AMA], 1959).

Butler's first scientific articles resulted from collaborative, cross-disciplinary work with Margolis, evaluating the benefits and risks of using chlorpromazine as a therapeutic intervention. Based on an evaluation of fifty-three patients treated for various psychiatric disorders with the drug, the pair (along with Butler's fellow resident, Ames Fischer, MD) reported that it "has been a common clinical experience" that chlorpromazine caused dermatitis. Symptoms ceased, however, when the medication stopped, raising questions among investigators and practitioners concerning whether the benefits outweighed the costs (Margolis, Butler, & Fischer, 1955). A year later Margolis, Fischer, and Butler (now joined by Alexander Simon) issued "clinical observations with chlorpromazine," based on findings initially reported at a symposium on psychopharmacology sponsored by the American Academy for the Advancement of Science (Kline, 1956).

While this article might seem to be merely one in a series of interesting papers issued by Langley Porter investigators on psychopharmacology, it is worth noting that its publication date coincided with a major jump in federal interest in mental illness. In 1955 Congress enacted the Mental Health Study Act, which called for "an objective, thorough, nationwide analysis and reevaluation of the human and economic problems of mental health." Debates erupted over whether experts should give precedence to promoting mental health over battling mental illness. The commission charged with data collection chose to define aims broadly (which, not surprisingly, raised a different set of turf issues). It sought expert opinions from the social and behavioral disciplines as well as the biomedical sciences for a "radical reconceptualization of the problems and possibly a reconstruction of the institutions so that resource-use might be more economical and mental health better served" (National Institutes of Health, 2010). From the survey emerged a ten-volume series, *Action for Mental Health* (1961), which served as the basis for John F. Kennedy's legislative action in this area. At the time NIH was underwriting 11,500 biomedical projects in universities and nonprofit institutions at a cost in excess of $250 million (Strickland, 1972:169). Langley Porter Psychiatric Institute benefited mightily from competing successfully over the augmented pool of federal dollars.

The publication on "chlorpromazine dermatitis" had professional consequences for Butler: it brought him to the attention of neuroscientist and physiologist Seymour S. Kety, MD, widely considered the father of biological psychiatry. (Kety not only discovered a method for measuring blood flow in the brain but in the 1960s offered evidence for the importance of genetic factors in schizophrenia.) In 1951 Kety had left a professorship at his alma mater, the University of Pennsylvania Medical School, for the National Institutes of Health (Harden 1986). His reputation as a basic scientist and intellectual leader impressed NIH recruiters, who promised him "free range to hire staff, an unrestricted budget, and beds" in Bethesda (Hannaway, 2008:43). NIH entrusted Kety, as scientific director, with designing intramural research programs and choosing laboratory chiefs for two new centers, the National Institute of Mental Health (NIMH) and the National Institute of Neurological Diseases and Blindness. He proposed laboratories for disciplines instead of diseases, earmarking biophysics, biochemistry, neurophysiology, (experimental) psychology, pharmacology, anatomy, experimental neuropathology, and socio-environmental studies. Intramural work at NIMH in the 1950s focused not just on bench science but also on behavioral and social-science research as well as clinical investigations (Holzman, 2000; Sokoloff, n.d.).

Butler interested Kety because of his work in psychopharmacology; both men had done studies on chlorpromazine. Butler immediately recognized the opportunities he would have if he joined Kety, who put a premium on excellence in basic science and cross-disciplinary researchers, however nontraditional their academic pedigrees. Kety later recalled:

I began to establish the organization of the Intramural Program of the NIMH and, also, to lay down the philosophy. I decided right off the bat that biology was going to be of considerable importance in psychiatry and in the study of mental illness, because I was convinced that the brain had a great deal to do with mental illness. . . . It was obvious that what we needed was a great deal of basic research. We needed much more information about fundamental aspects of the processes, the biological processes of the brain, before we could even think of attacking the practical problems. . . . We had to firm up the knowledge of basic information about the brain and we had to firm up our knowledge of the mental illnesses itself before we could upgrade the cross between them.

(HANNAWAY, 2008; KOPIN, 1995:10)

During a two-hour interview, walking the hills of San Francisco, the men hammered out details for an appointment. (Butler's other option was to stay in the Bay Area and work at Alcatraz investigating the criminal mind.) Kety promised to give Butler freedom to pursue what he wished, a luxury he would not have been accorded on a university's tenure track. Furthermore, Kety could protect the young investigator from intramural rivalries in NIMH's Clinical Lab (Hannaway, 2008).

Because of the time it took to complete the security clearances in order to affiliate with NIMH, Butler sought a temporary post once he had completed his first year of psychiatric residency at Langley Porter. He was hired as a physician in an outpatient clinic in a Kaiser Permanente Hospital in San Francisco, which became a model for health maintenance organizations (HMOs). Kaiser Permanente offered prepaid group practice, so the job gave Butler an important lens with which to look at medical economics.

MULTIDISCIPLINARY BREAKTHROUGHS AT NIMH

Upon Butler's arrival at NIMH, Kety immediately put him on an internal committee to decide how best to spend an additional allocation of $1.5 million to study tranquilizers. Besides contributing to debates over psychopharmacology's validity in treating mental illness, Butler joined NIMH's Laboratory of Clinical Sciences' investigations into mechanisms of actions associated with tranquilizers.

In addition, Butler had to complete his three-year residency to become board certified in psychiatry. Only one of his three years at Langley Porter counted toward this end, and Kety gave him credit for a second year based on his work at NIMH. To round out the residency, Butler spent a year on the staff at Chestnut Lodge, a tertiary-care psychiatric unit in nearby Rockville, Maryland, where 60 percent of the self-paying patients stayed under care for two years (Judd & McGlashan, 2003; McGlashan & Fenton, 1998). Physicians, who rarely prescribed psychoactive drugs, offered fifty-minute psychoanalytic sessions four or five times a week. Butler treated four schizophrenic patients and established an experimental psychotherapy unit.

In 1956 NIMH—in partnership with the National Academy of Sciences, the National Research Council, and the American Psychiatric Association—sponsored a multidisciplinary conference on problems of evaluation in psychopharmacology, which NIMH director Robert Felix, MD, cheekily described as an "exchange of ignorance. . . . I think that everyone would agree that we really knew pitifully little about the effects of drugs on behavior and maybe even less about their use in mental illness" (Cole & Gerard, 1959:v). With Edward Evarts, MD, then head of the physiology section of NIMH's Clinical Lab, Butler presented a review of the effects of chlorpromazine and reserpine (a second drug that he had analyzed at Langley Porter). The pair highlighted the drugs' effects and benefits and then compared them with other therapies as reported in various controlled studies. While acknowledging that researchers credited chlorpromazine and reserpine with improving patients' rapport and communication, Evarts and Butler claimed that "we are not about to have illusions about our first experiences with these new medications." They felt that the effectiveness of psychotherapy (with or without pharmacological adjuncts) was difficult to measure (Cole & Gerard, 1959:76).

In an unrelated move, Kety proposed that several staff join him in undergoing didactic psychoanalysis to determine how much valance should be accorded Freudian theories in the work at NIMH. Accepting Kety's invitation, Butler worked with Dr. Leslie Farber, an existential psychotherapist (Farber, 1966). Through analysis Butler retrieved memories about his grandfather. In addition, Farber brought Jewish theologian Martin Buber to Washington, whom Butler greatly admired. The work with Farber positioned Butler for an eventual appointment at the Washington School of Psychiatry.

Butler's arrival at NIMH coincided with a major expansion in NIH's aims. "Knowledge of life processes and of phenomena underlying health and disease is still grossly inadequate," observed NIH director James Shannon, who continued:

> In the absence of broad general theory, such as exists in the physical sciences, the development of diagnostic, therapeutic, and preventive capability will continue to be dependent upon empirical approaches, serendipity, and the intuitive brilliance of too few gifted individuals. Therefore, the hope of major advances lies in sustaining broad and free-ranging inquiry into all aspects of the phenomena of life, limited only by the criteria of excellence, the scientific importance, and the seriousness and competence of the investigators.
>
> (SHANNON, 1967:104–5)

The advance of Big Science at the National Institutes of Health depended on first-rate researchers, who were well trained in their respective disciplines. Those who made their careers at NIH generally enjoyed involving themselves in big, multidisciplinary projects. They were intent on understanding and alleviating major challenges related to health and disease, regardless (within the limits of a chief's approval) of the cost and time required to accomplish scientific objectives. That this approach to making science proved wildly successful, Butler pointed out to me, greatly influenced his attitudes about institution building when he later assumed a leadership role at NIH.

Butler spent the next eight years on a team project that integrated biological, medical, social-psychological, and statistical bases of healthy aging. Besides the articles that grew out of that landmark project, NIMH published a monograph, *Human Aging*. Looking back, Butler told me that he considered his involvement in interdisciplinary research and dissemination, which culminated in the publication of *Human Aging*, to be the most intellectually stimulating phase of his career. Others shared his enthusiasm. "Many efforts at collaboration prove abortive or, if carried through, are poorly productive, since each participant feels he has sacrificed an important tenet in the interests of a common goal which is deprecated thereby," observed Robert A. Cohen, MD, director of NIMH's clinical investigations, in his preface to *Human Aging*. "Here is a report from some investigators who triumphed over these natural secessionists and isolationist tendencies, were gradually molded into a group and who, in my opinion, have set forth an interesting and somewhat unique product" (Cohen, 1963:ix–x).

Cohen's description of the NIMH team of researchers producing a "somewhat unique product" is accurate, for there was only one other group of multidisciplinary researchers seeking to distinguish healthy and pathological aspects of growing older. In 1955, under the leadership of Ewald Busse (a psychiatrist), a team at Duke University launched a survey of normal aging. Noteworthy for their inclusion of African American subjects, Duke psychiatrists obtained electroencephalograms on cortical activities and tested elders' attitudes toward such issues as children, retirement, and guilt (Achenbaum & Albert, 1995:60; Busse et al., 1954; Silverman, Busse, & Barnes, 1955).

Of the twenty-two investigators, five (including Butler) served as coeditors of *Human Aging*. Cohen noted that "Birren and the associates in his section were the only ones who had devoted any considerable portion of their scientific careers to the study of aging" (1963:x). James Birren joined the Public Health Service in 1947, where he worked with Nathan W. Shock in the Gerontology Unit. Three years later he moved to NIMH; there he created the first section on aging in the institutes (Achenbaum & Albert, 1995:37–38). Samuel W. Greenhouse, when not providing statistical designs and analyses for *Human Aging*, served as an adviser and reviewer for several agencies outside NIH, including the U.S. Public Health Service and the Federal Aviation Agency Council of Epidemiologic Methodology Committee. Louis Sokoloff, MD, a student of Seymour Kety's, joined the venture to learn more about brain circulation and metabolism in a segment of the population he had not studied. Prior to this collaboration, Sokoloff had demonstrated his ability to meld neuroscience and biological chemistry others taught him at NIMH (Squire, 2011). Child psychologist Dr. Marian Yarrow, whose *They Learn What They Live* (1952) was cited in *Brown*

v. *Board of Education of Topeka*, ran NIMH's developmental psychology laboratory (Hevesi, 2007). Yarrow wanted to investigate aspects of growth and decline at the other end of the life course.

"This study began in 1955 with a focus on the interrelations between cerebral physiological changes of advancing age and psychological capacities and psychiatric symptoms," the co-editors noted in the introduction (Birren et al., 1963:2). The *Human Aging* project evolved and expanded over time as investigators pursued new ideas and examined each other's findings. At the outset the investigators were predisposed to challenge the dominant, scientific motif of aging-as-decline (Achenbaum, 1978, 1995). The few important works in medical aspects of senescence had made an orthodoxy out of this theme. In modern times it began with Jean-Martin Charcot's *Clinical Lectures on the Diseases of Old Age* (1881), based on studies of localized lesions among inmates at the Salpêtrière Hospital in Paris. A few decades later Nobel laureate Elie Metchnikoff went further than Charcot and declared that "old age, then, is an infectious, chronic disease, which is manifested by a degeneration" (1903:548). As late as 1939 Edmund V. Cowdry's august contributors accentuated the problems of aging more than its potentialities. The challenge facing the NIMH team of researchers and clinicians was to create a research design that permitted examination of a representative sample of older people since they knew that "many prevailing ideas and facts about aging and the aged come from studies of the sick and institutionalized" (Birren et al., 1963:1).

Human Aging meant to disaggregate the effects of disease from "normal" processes of aging. Researchers faced a daunting challenge because so little was known about basic processes and mechanisms of growing older; no one associated with the multidisciplinary project was prepared to define aging as a "single pacemaker which controls change in a broad range of anatomical, physiological, and psychological characteristics" (Cohen, 1963:2; see also Achenbaum, 1978; Achenbaum & Albert, 1995; Nascher, 1914). The co-editors of *Human Aging* decided that it would be premature to generate grand hypotheses about senescence, despite their curiosity about several potential interdependencies. The NIMH team realized that more research had to be undertaken before elucidating systems of integration and patterns of control at the social, psychological, or biochemical levels. Free to work independently, the group proved remarkably cohesive. "During the 5 years of this project, a continuous research seminar operated"; then, for three additional years, the editorial committee collaborated in conceptualizing ideas about age and aging, followed by interpreting the data for dissemination" (Birren et al., 1963:3).

Human Aging was a modest, cross-sectional project compared to present-day benchmark gerontological studies. The pilot study was not representative: from an initial pool of fifty-four, investigators chose forty-seven men, largely recruited from the Philadelphia area and the District of Columbia, drawing from the National Association of Retired Civil Service Employees. Subjects ranged in years from sixty-five to ninety-one; seventy-one was the median age. In terms of education, income, and living conditions, the sample was generally better off than the population at large. Since securing a healthful sample was critical to fulfilling the aims of *Human Aging,* the participants selected for the study were in better condition than most men their ages. Twenty-seven subjects (Group I) were deemed "optimally healthy for their age" on the basis of eight screenings, including cardiovascular and pulmonary tests; among the rest (Group II) the presence of "disease was minimal and asymptomatic" (14). Once the prescreening was completed, the research team performed physical and neurological exams, blood studies, urinalyses, electrocardiograms, x-rays, and other tests of ventilator function, vital signs, and physical measurements on volunteer subjects over the two-week period that they spent in NIH's Clinical Center.

Group reports constitute most of *Human Aging.* Greenhouse explained the overall research design, acknowledging restrictions on the robustness of statistical methods for multiple testing across behavioral and biomedical domains. In "Medical Investigation of the Processes of Aging," Leslie Libow underscored a theme that recurred throughout the study: there were marked physiological differences between Groups I and II. On the basis of disciplinary-specific analyses, the researchers who prepared the next five chapters addressed intergroup differences and similarities in test results between the project's two subsets. Different sets of investigators measured metabolism, cerebral circulation, motor abilities and psychomotor responses, electroencephalograms, and auditory perception and developed a battery of thirty-two variables to assess mental and perceptual tests in late life. Occasionally they made passing references comparing test results of Groups I and II with those of younger people; no consistent trend emerges.

Butler and his immediate supervisor at NIMH, Seymour Perlin, MD, prepared the longest chapter, a fifty-eight-page analysis of "Psychiatric Aspects of Adaptation to the Aging Experience." Like those that preceded it, this contribution begins by underscoring the need to recognize that the "emotionally-disturbed, community-resident aged rarely receive psychiatric treatment" (159). Among other things, the pair wanted to determine if psychotherapy or other psychiatric interventions helped elderly persons who were impeded by a chronic ailment or loneliness but not afflicted by any debilitating mental disorder. Avowedly multidisciplinary in their pursuit of empirical and theoretical knowledge, Perlin and Butler issued an analysis dense in data. More than was apparent in other chapters, Perlin and Butler presented lengthy case studies, citing publications by mentors (such as Karl Bowman) and rising analysts (such as Erik Erikson).

Three subjects give a sense of their sample. Case 24, orphaned at an early age, shuttled from foster home to foster home. In adulthood he made a pretense of performing expected family and marital roles. Retirement caused an identity crisis, exacerbated by the departure of his children from home (176). Perlin and Butler diagnosed case 54 as a seventy-two-year-old who adapted well to a schizoid personality with obsessive and compulsive features. This former political science professor viewed his coming of age "scientifically," by denying losses and leaving behind interpersonal skills (180). Case 57 was a seventy-four-year-old retired widower with low morale but no manifest disorder. The loss of his mother and five siblings in youth predisposed him to a state of isolation evident in interviews. This was the first man of the pool to die after the study, Perlin and Butler reported (182). Such subjects enabled the researches to get inside senescence, to "explore *with* [a subject] his aging experience and his adaptation to it" (160). The pair claimed that their interviews with subjects, directed and open-ended for two to three hours in length, were "rarely dull."

Perlin and Butler's bottom line in "Psychiatric Aspects of Adaptation to the Aging Experience" was that chronological age was a less reliable predictor of psychiatric states in Groups I and II than were personality traits, losses, and diseases. They found that nearly a fifth of the subjects were mildly depressed; diagnosable illnesses were caused by external stresses, not by aging processes or physical impairment. The meanings and significance that older people placed on psychosocial losses and disruptions, the pair discovered, were as important as the nature and frequency of those stressors in late-life adaptation. This led Perlin and Butler to conclude that "maintenance of a functional sense of identity seemed to be crucial to successful adaptation" (Neugarten, 1968:239). If so, it followed that there was a "need for revision in assessment and diagnosis with the aged" (Birren et al., 1963:188–89). This essay anticipated themes that would be enunciated in a concluding chapter on "Interdisciplinary Relationships."

The next three essays added further detailed information and cross-disciplinary perspectives to the empirical findings that Perlin and Butler reported about mental well-being in later years. Margaret Thaler Singer's "Personality Measurements in the Aged" found scores for verbal behavior and an ability to follow test directions more similar between Group I and younger subjects than between the sample's two subsets. According to Conan Kornetsky, the Minnesota Multiphasic Personality Inventory, although rarely used heretofore to study normal aged populations, confirmed Perlin and Butler's description of manifestations of depression found among subjects in Group II. The report on "Social Psychological Characteristics of Old Age" by Marian Yarrow's group began with a warning that generalizations were difficult, given the state of gerontological knowledge. Too little was known theoretically and empirically, Yarrow's lab claimed, about antecedents and consequences of "the gross settings in which the aged person lives, such as institution or community, retired status or not retired, one social class or ethnic culture or another" (160). Citing scholars such as Gordon Strieb and Peter Townsend, Yarrow and associates stressed that retirement gradually engulfed late life and generally augmented the importance of family in these subjects' lives. The essay ended tentatively: without a richer conceptual framework at their disposal, investigators had to wait for longitudinal data in order to capture whatever causal, temporal dimension might exist.

Birren, Butler, Greenhouse, Sokoloff, and Yarrow devoted two chapters to wrapping up *Human Aging*. They began with "Interdisciplinary Relationships: Interrelations of Physiological, Psychological, and Psychiatric Findings, in Health, Elderly Men." They acknowledged that "interconnections among the medical, cerebral circulatory, metabolic, and EEG variables revealed few statistically significant correlations" (293), though five years of research had yielded 198 possible correlations between psychological and physiological measurements among subjects. Noting that that number represents more factors than (they speculated) would be required to assess the young, they emphasized "the need to probe further into the physiological as well as the environmental basis for late life decline in psychomotor speed and in mental ability shown by some individuals or alternatively to search for the bases for the maintenance of high level capacities" (311). Insofar as depression and slowing of reaction times occur in younger people, they deduced, this was proof that something besides the inexorable passage of time affects human aging. Hence "it is important to discover and recognize those factors which are not necessarily inevitably or unalterably part of the aging process but are subject to preventive and therapeutic measures" (300).

The co-editors challenged images of age widespread in the early 1960s that portrayed humans declining in later years into a disease-ridden state of self-absorbed disengagement, of men dozing in rocking chairs or stooped over canes. Instead, the NIMH team offered an optimistic portrait of human aging in their summary and conclusions. "The healthy aged were found to have disorders, evolving from personality and life experience, which appear similar to those affecting the young" (314). Physical, pathological, and psychological conditions varied among NIMH subjects in Groups I and II. Because it was not yet possible to rank order the effects of genes, personality types, propensity for chronic maladies or mental illness, or environmental conditions, the NIMH researchers underscored the great need for systematic studies of the mechanisms and processes of aging to explicate the social-psychological and biomedical factors that shaped human adaptability:

When one is faced with the broad range of behavioral and neural changes of aging, it is difficult to keep the details in balanced emphasis. In discussing the present results one would like to retain the surety surrounding the study of isolated variables, yet there is equally the scientific motivation to consider the survival and behavior of the organism as an integrated phenomenon. The interrelatedness of the manifestations of aging remains a tentative matter.

(315; SEE ALSO BUTLER, DASTOR, & PERLIN, 1965)

While the tone of this and other passages is measured, Birren and his co-editors persisted nonetheless in accentuating the positive implications of their cross-disciplinary research: "With the promise of medical advances in the control of the now common metabolic diseases of later life, more individuals will be seen who are old in years but functionally young by present standards." Human aging, in their opinion, demanded "increased study of interpersonal relations and the environmental elements in optimum personality development over the life span" (316).

Wanting to go a step further, Butler proceeded to publish interpretive summaries of his own. He recast the interdisciplinary features of *Human Aging* in one of his oft-cited articles, "The Façade of Chronological Age," in a way that he hoped would be *"of particular interest to the psychiatrist."* So "much of the literature concerning the aged and aging had heretofore derived principally from studies of the sick and institutionalized. . . . Little appeared to be known about healthy and social autonomous aging. We knew that certain cultural stereotypes affected the contemporary picture of the aged and the process of aging" (Neugarten, 1968:235–42). True to the spirit of the NIMH report, Butler took care not to adduce conclusions about physical, physiological, psychological, and social processes that went beyond findings validated at NIMH. He reiterated a central finding of *Human Aging*: Growing older did not unfold through a homeostatic process or synchronous manner. Butler and his colleagues were examining "vigorous, candid, interesting . . . resourceful and optimistic" elderly males, who were "quite different from and superior to other samples of aged persons that have been previously described." Butler reframed the project's aim to address a "broad screening question" (his words) in order to sharpen the current and future purview of gerontological inquiry: "How might we disentangle the contributions of disease, social losses, preexisting personality, and the like from changes that might more properly be regarded as age-specific?" (Neugarten, 1968:238).

Butler highlighted for mental-health professionals various correlations across and within disciplinary findings from *Human Aging*. He specified measurement changes in blood circulation, cognition, and psychosocial conditions that he and his colleagues suspected might contribute to depression in late life. In addition, he informed psychiatrists that diseases (such as arteriosclerosis), auditory and visual defects, and social isolation all colored evaluations and treatments of mental disorders. That health-care professionals labor under too many misconceptions about human aging, indicated Butler, compounds the problem in caring for older persons:

> As a consequence of a careful multidisciplinary pilot study, we have found evidence to suggest that many manifestations heretofore associated with aging per se reflect instead medical illness, personality variables, and social-cultural effects. . . . Intensive studies . . . would contribute to our understanding of the subjective experience of aging and approaching death (Butler, 1960; 1963). Longitudinal studies, of course, would enhance our opportunities of classifying changes as to whether they are age-specific, disease-linked, *etc.* If we can get beyond the façade of chronological aging we open up the possibility of modification through both prevention and treatment.
>
> (NEUGARTEN, 1968:242; SEE ALSO BUSSE ET AL., 1954; FRAZIER, HOOKER, & SIEGLER, 1993; SILVERMAN, BUSSE, & BARNES, 1955)

Without deviating from the purposes or distorting the empirical results of the NIMH study, Butler in "The Façade of Chronological Age" deliberately staked a claim for his right to identify as a geriatrician and gerontologist— something that his superiors had not certified when the young psychiatrist arrived at NIMH. Citing his prior work that contributed to his involvement with *Human Aging*, he underscored how much basic and applied research and how many large and small projects and disciplinary-specific as well as cross-disciplinary inquiries had to be undertaken. And he made clear that not all the important work in gerontology would be executed in institutions and laboratories. Mental-health professionals had services, including therapy, to offer older men and women who were enjoying healthful, well-adjusted lives in the community.

What did Butler gain from participating in NIMH's project? He was more convinced than ever that the first aim of gerontological research was to remove the distorting masks of aging. Scientists and practitioners had to develop theories and interventions that took account of the diverse, subjective experiences of growing older. "In our lifetime (if at all) it is not likely that the inexorable processes of aging will be amenable to human intervention," he concluded, "but it cannot be too greatly emphasized that it is necessary to be able to recognize those factors which are open to change" (Birren et al., 1963:242). At the end of his tenure at the National Institute of Mental Health, Butler committed himself to piercing the façade of chronological age through multidisciplinary research. Seasoned through his editorial work on the *Columbia Daily Spectator*, the physician intended to communicate through important media outlets breakthroughs in ways that science and technology could improve the quality of late life for ordinary people.

In retrospect, Butler seemed poised to engage in professional domains where he had not received specialized training, displaying talents not yet tested. By engaging in politics and policy making in the nation's capital, he would learn how to undermine negative images of age and aging, which were strongly held by health-care professionals and the American public. Butler was ready to collaborate with others to create programs to alleviate suffering and maximize capabilities in later years.

four
FORGING WASHINGTON CONNECTIONS

Between 1963 and 1975, from his departure from the National Institute of Mental Health to his start at the National Institute on Aging (NIA), Butler benefited greatly from living and working in Washington, D.C. During this period he coined the term "ageism" and wrote *Why Survive? Being Old in America*, for which he won a Pulitzer Prize. He earned respect as a smart, compassionate, and versatile physician with a knack for advocacy. His sudden metamorphosis from professional apprentice to gerontological insider caught even Butler by surprise. After all, he was primarily a practicing psychiatrist who supplemented his income by teaching health-care professionals. Yet his other extracurricular activities—serving on local commissions and joining boards of Washington-based groups advocating for senior citizens—brought him to the attention of individuals who would assist him in addressing and ameliorating old-age problems for the rest of his career.

Supporters in journalism, on Capitol Hill, and in advocacy circles emboldened Butler, in a period of social activism, to become a tenacious champion for older people. Shocked and angered by the extent of elder abuse (physical, psychological, and social) in the nation's capital, he made a reputation for himself through proposing sensible solutions to inequities and injustice. By 1976, when he officially took over as NIA's founding director, Robert Butler's name and phone number were well-known to many members of the media. Prominent Washingtonians with a stake in the aging enterprise viewed him as a reliable ally, a health-care professional who was unafraid of "speaking truth to power" (Wildavsky, 1979). He could persuade idea brokers and citizens with his presence and voice.

BECOMING PROMINENT IN THE DISTRICT OF COLUMBIA

In 1961, prior to leaving NIMH, Butler joined the Washington School of Psychiatry (WSP). He intermittently was a clinical associate professor of medicine at Howard and George Washington universities. At WSP he served as a research psychiatrist and gerontologist at the Study Center from 1962 until 1976. Despite the school's frequently shaky financial situation (Ozarin, 1999; Rioch, 1985), it was an obvious position for the thirty-four-year-old psychiatrist to accept. Dr. Leslie Farber, Butler's analyst during the tour of duty at NIMH, had become WSP's head five years earlier. He launched the Forum on Psychiatry and the Humanities at the school. Chestnut Lodge physicians and other local health professionals participated in seminars and courses (Coles, 1967; Judd & McGlashan, 2003; Rioch, 1986).

Butler encountered a different sort of cross-disciplinary interplay at WSP than he had experienced at Langley Porter Psychiatric Institute or the National Institute of Mental Health (Butler & Sullivan, 1963). Colleagues at the Washington School of Psychiatry incorporated materials from the humanities and qualitative social sciences into their lectures on psychoanalysis and psychiatry. Butler was receptive to such cross-disciplinary fertilization.

Some of Butler's WSP associates were helpful mentors. Notable in this regard was Robert Maynard (1937–93), who became the first African American to serve as a national newspaper correspondent and editorial member of the *Washington Post*. (In 1977 he left Washington, D.C., to teach at Berkeley; six years later he acquired the *Oakland Tribune* from the Gannett Company.) Besides enjoying each other's company, the pair respected the media's power to convey ideas robust enough to change minds. Maynard paved the way for Butler to meet reporters and editors at the *Washington Post* and the *New York Times* as well as Washington correspondents for *Newsweek* and *Time*. He also introduced Butler to journalist Peter Weaver, who was willing to do four public-television shows until Butler's voice cracked from nervousness. Maynard and Butler team-taught a seminar on "Man as a Political Animal" at WSP; they invited notables in the District of Columbia to help focus each evening's discussion on topics such as power, leadership, or community. Maynard served as a key adviser during Butler's years at the National Institute on Aging.

Butler told me that he and Maynard became very close friends and neighbors. The pair ran together. Maynard married Nancy Hicks in Butler's home. Butler flew to the West Coast frequently to see his friend, especially when he was dying of prostate cancer. Maynard's son and grandson were at Butler's deathbed; his daughter, Dori, delivered a eulogy at Butler's memorial.

Furthermore, Butler became increasingly involved in the Group for the Advancement of Psychiatry (GAP) during his tenure at the Washington School of Psychiatry. GAP challenged what its members considered outmoded etiologies and treatments of mental disorders; often they targeted practices endorsed by the fairly staid American Psychiatric Association. In addition, consistent with the activist stance that GAP presented in *The Social Responsibility of Psychiatry, a Statement of Orientation*, it addressed controversial psychosocial issues (Group for the Advancement of Psychiatry, 1950; see also 1954, 1955, 1957). Through GAP, psychoanalyst Judd Marmor befriended Butler. One-time president of both the American Psychiatric Association and GAP, Dr. Marmor advocated group psychotherapy and short-term behavioral therapies with traditional psychodynamic approaches, of which Butler approved (Hausman, 2004).

Butler's practice conformed to standards customary at the time. He worked out of his home, at 3815 Huntington Street, seeing patients in fifty-minute sessions on weekdays from 7:30 A.M. to 7:00 P.M. and on Saturdays from 8:00 A.M. until 1:00 P.M. Unlike his peers, who typically specialized in treating a certain mental disorder or worked with particular segments of the population, or both, Butler enjoyed working with adolescents (with whom he took walks during sessions) as well as older people (whom he would visit at home, meeting over kitchen tables). "He was a fine shrink and a kind loving man. He had a way of getting to the heart of things, sometimes quite sarcastically," recalled commentator, actor, and lawyer Ben Stein (2010).

While he had been trained to employ psychodynamic approaches, Butler gradually departed from standard practices. As we saw in chapter 1, during the 1960s and 1970s he refined his conceptualization and execution of the life review so patients could make sense of late-life reminiscences. In 1970 he developed a professional relationship with Myrna I. Lewis (1938–2005), a graduate of Columbia's School of Social Work. The pair over the next five years conducted four age-integrated psychotherapy groups, with eight to ten members, ranging in age from fifteen to eighty. The participants that Lewis and Butler selected, while not psychotic, generally were undergoing a life crisis associated with adolescence, relationships, work or retirement, or impending death. "Such groups are concerned not only with intrinsic psychiatric disorders but with preventive and remedial treatment of people as they pass through the usual vicissitudes of the life cycle" (Butler, 1974:535). It was helpful for transference, the pair concluded, that as co-therapists they differed in gender and discipline, "to provide a psychodynamic and sociological orientation for each group" (Butler & Lewis, 1982:331).

THE BEGINNING OF POLITICAL ACTIVISM

Butler maintained links, intellectual and personal, with associates after he left the National Institute of Mental Health. He published follow-up materials from his work at NIMH on *Human Aging* (see Butler, Dastor, & Perlin, 1974:229–38). He kept in touch with former co-investigator Louis Sokoloff and his wife, Barbara. In addition, he deepened his professional and personal ties with Dexter Means Bullard Jr., MD, who in 1969 succeeded his father as medical director of Chestnut Lodge, where Butler had completed his psychiatry residency. Butler recalled that conversations with Bullard and Maynard heightened his frustration, which began during his internship, with the gap that he discerned between the aims of psychiatry and the search for solutions to real-life problems. He was taught neither the connection between patients' health and their psychological outlooks nor the pertinence of power or anger in social relations. Racial divisions in America, not surprisingly, deeply disturbed him.

Others shared Butler's disillusionment. The nation's second Civil Rights movement was galvanizing fundamental political and policy changes in the Capitol and state houses. It transformed daily interactions between blacks and whites. Witnessing considerable racial blindness in standard psychiatric practices, Butler became interested in mental-health issues affecting minority youth who came from stable home environments. As we shall see, he also helped to create institutional structures to respond to the plight of older blacks (see Bullard et al., 1967; Glaser et al., 1968).

Integral to Butler's ongoing self-education was his ability to build on intellectual capital as he developed new ideas and strategies for engagement. This is evident in his article "Aspects of Survival and Adaptation in Human Aging" (1967). There Butler offered his own interpretation of a five-year, follow-up analysis on *Human Aging*'s subjects conducted in NIMH's Clinical Center, which he characterized as "one of the first comprehensive longitudinal studies of medically healthy, community-resident older people in which the multidisciplinary approach is utilized." Thirty-nine of the forty-seven men in the original study had survived; three had entered a nursing home; none was being treated in a psychiatric institution. "As a whole, they remained as before: vigorous, flexible, and resourceful," observed Butler. "Supporting data were found for the hypothesis that . . . older people universally undergo a life review leading to various preparations for loss, bodily dissolution, and death" (1242). The decision to disseminate a perspective that went beyond the NIMH script was not an act of defiance. Rather, it signaled Butler's maturation as a clinician: he reviewed earlier NIMH data through the lens of his work with community-based, "healthy" elders as well as insights with clients approaching death.

Butler's growing reputation in Washington as a political activist brought opportunities to change older patients' conditions and treatment in nursing homes. In 1959, in a speech before a group of nursing-home owners in Maryland, he argued that health-care professionals and the public at large held stereotypic and depressing images of institutionalized elders:

[The old man] is the picture of mental and physical failure. He has lost and cannot replace friends, spouse, jobs, status, power, influence, income. . . . His body shrinks; so, too, does the flow of blood to his brain. His mind does not utilize oxygen and sugar at the same rate as formerly. Feeble, uninteresting, he awaits his death, a burden to society, to his family, and to himself.

(BUTLER, 1974:531)

To alter this "caricature of a lifelong personality," based on the 5 percent of older Americans (according to the 1950 census) residing in institutions, declared Butler, required hard data on the attributes, capacities, and social integration of those successfully aging in the community.

Butler began to test his hunches about how rehabilitation might improve the environments where older people lived. In the 1960s he helped to start an adult day center in the basement of the Baptist Home for the Aged in Washington. "It was amazing to see people who were bedfast or chairfast come alive with the opportunity to mix with other people, and this enlivened the home's residents, as well," Butler recalled. "They benefitted in other ways, too. Psychotropic drug usage, for example, declined markedly" (Peck, 1996).

In 1968 Butler was contacted by Claire Townsend and five other recent graduates of Miss Porter's School, an elite independent school for women. Together with one of their teachers, the so-called Maiden Muckrakers had decided to investigate the financing and conditions in nursing homes instead of spending summer vacations with their peers. To gain advice, support, and credibility, the young ladies invited individuals with potentially useful ideas and contacts to their Washington townhouse for a home-cooked meal. Butler accepted their invitation. He "stayed past midnight, a fount of tips and leads and other useful pieces of information" (Martin,

2002:102; see Marcello, 2004:57). Seeking both experience and exposure, like the Maiden Muckrakers, Butler agreed to work with Ms. Townsend, who became project director of Ralph Nader's Study Group Report on Nursing Homes. The teenagers gathered interviews with residents and staff, visited nursing home, and kept detailed journals. From this material emerged a report worthy of Nader's Raiders, *Old Age: The Last Segregation*, which appeared in hardback in 1969 and in paperback two years later (Townsend, 1971).

Claire Townsend and her colleagues recommended greater oversight of nursing homes, better professional education, and fuller consumer protection. *Old Age* helped to spark a wave of exposes into the quality of life for institutionalized elders. To defuse the scandal, the Maryland affiliate of the American Nursing Home Association placed a full-page ad in November 1970 in the *Baltimore Sun* inviting readers "to see with your own eyes the accomplishments that have been made in the care and treatment of the people whom we call . . . our guests." Yet management declined access to the Harbor View Nursing and Convalescence Center when Butler and William Hutton, executive director of the National Council of Senior Citizens, arrived unannounced to inspect the site (Butler, 1975b:283–85; see also Achenbaum, 1986:22, 27; Carleton, 1873:51, 57;Trattner, 1974:54).

The controversy surrounding the Nader report piqued the interest of Sen. Frank Moss (D-UT), who held hearings on long-term care in December 1970. Claire Townsend testified, as did William Hutton. Butler also testified, claiming that older people in community facilities in and around Washington, D.C., endured worse conditions than typically found in nursing homes (Butler, 1971a:139–41, 1971b:197–201; United States Senate, 1971).

After the Maiden Muckrakers matriculated in universities and colleges, Butler continued to seek improvements in the quality of nursing homes. He worked closely with Val Halamandaris, who began his Washington career as an aide to Senator Moss (1962–1969) before becoming associate counsel to the U.S. Senate Special Committee on Aging (1969–1978). Accompanied by *CBS News*'s Barry Sarafin, in 1973 Butler and Halamandaris paid an unscheduled visit to a nursing home outside of Pittsburgh, which was known for its filth, odors, and poor standards for care. Butler told me that the smell of coffee greeting the investigative team did not deter Halaman-daris from subpoenaing access to records, which indicated that the opera-tors, having been tipped off, hired extra aides a few days before to clean up the residents and their surroundings.

This, among other investigations, became the crux of the Senate Special Committee on Aging's 1974 hearings on "Nursing Home Care in the United States: Failure in Public Policy," at which Butler testified. The testi-monies revealed that (1) nursing homes were not adhering to Medicaid regulations enacted in 1967; (2) despite a high incidence of psychopathol-ogy, nursing-home patients received little psychiatric treatment and mini-mal physical care, from ill-trained aides at understaffed sites; and (3) there were "numerous examples of cruelty, negligence, danger from fires, food poisoning, virulent infections, lack of human dignity, callousness and un-necessary regulation" (Butler, 1975a:897). Such conditions led Halaman-daris to denounce intermediate-care facilities as "the universal receptacle of the unwanted" (Butler, 1975b:294). Butler urged greater flexibility in designating how federal dollars were spent on long-term care; those cur-rently in an institutional setting, he opined, might do better physically and mentally if they resided at home assisted by families (Butler, 1975a:897).

Butler joined members of the Group for the Advancement of Psychiatry in addressing another facet of custodial care for older adults who were suf-fering from mental illness. As a result of incentives under the Mental Health Act of 1956, which encouraged deinstitutionalization of residents, the population in U.S. mental hospitals had roughly fallen from 500,000 to 337,000 between 1955 and 1972. Concerned that many relocations amounted to "dumping" vulnerable people into nursing homes as well as into understaffed and resource-poor community mental-health centers, GAP issued a report on the "Crisis in Psychiatric Hospitalization." Dr. Jack Weinberg, elucidating GAP's position in testimony before a 1971 hearing of the U.S. Senate Special Committee on Aging, for which Butler served as a consultant, declared that "many of our mental institutions, though some of them may be snake pits, are better places than some of the nursing homes in view of the fact that they, at least, have such necessary items of care as 24-hour coverage by a nurse, a fire alarm system and the food in the State hospitals is nutritionally adequate" (Butler, 1974b:240–46; see also "Jack Weinberg," 1983:1239).

Sharing Weinberg's view that "the concept of community care for the chronically mentally ill [was] valuable but limited," Butler advocated that residences be upgraded to become total-care facilities with a full range of state-of-the-art medical, nursing, psychiatric, and social services (Achenbaum & Albert, 1995:93). Hotels, he opined, often were preferable to nursing homes and mental-health institutions as residential settings for elders.

Rethinking medical choices for older Americans, in Butler's view, would redirect how health-care professionals delineated, assessed, and executed elder care: "Clearly society, and its instruments, medicine and psychiatry, cannot discharge their responsibilities for the study, evaluation, care and treatment of chronic mental illness and the disorders of late life if old people are sequestered outside the mainstream of American medicine and psychiatry" (Butler, 1970:260). This sentence foreshadows Butler's three-pronged approach toward old-age policy making—a position he would maintain for the rest of his career. First, policy makers, health professionals, and the public had to stop marginalizing elderly individuals. Second, U.S. society was obliged, for the sake of justice, to give older citizens access to the best care possible. Third, to achieve these first two objectives would necessitate a radical restructuring of health care to guarantee everybody's common stake in growing older in a healthful manner.

Butler reached out to the Gerontological Society of America (GSA), founded in 1945. He already had a good working relationship with James Birren, who had assumed leadership at home and abroad partly through GSA connections. In 1966, attending the International Congress in Gerontology in Vienna, Butler was introduced to Ewald Busse, whose studies on aging at Duke he had followed while working on *Human Aging*. He also met Dr. Bernice Neugarten, who became one of GSA's intellectual giants and Butler's lifelong friend. Butler remembered fondly the term he spent teaching at the University of Chicago. He also recalled being snowbound with Neugarten and Birren in Neugarten's penthouse. The three plotted ways to transform research and teaching in aging through GSA. They wanted to reframe academic work in gerontology by stressing lifespan perspectives on late life.

The work done during that blizzard in Chicago reveals much about gerontology's three brightest stars and the state of the field in the late 1960s. In independent conversations, Neugarten, Birren, and Butler each told me that their confinement occasioned one of the intellectual highlights of their careers. All felt, as a result of this summit, that they could change gerontology's trajectory—long before any had hit stride. Neugarten surely was the most gifted theorist of the three, and Birren the most nimble academic architect. Butler surpassed the others in his ability to translate ideas in the media, thereby influencing possible ways to restructure the health-care delivery system and geriatric research; more than the others, he became a public persona.

For all their enthusiasm and sagacity, it must be noted that the field of aging in 1968 was small. Birren, Neugarten, and Butler could wield clout within gerontological circles without making waves beyond their spheres of influence. A lack of researchers, practitioners, and vocal constituency limited gerontology's impact on Big Science and the marketplace of ideas as a whole. At that moment in U.S. history, pundits and policy makers took notice of African Americans, women, and other disenfranchised groups, not older people.

CIVIC ENGAGEMENT

Throughout his career Robert Butler generously gave time to voluntary associations. Many of his endeavors reflected his desire to empower Americans of all ages, especially senior citizens, to enrich their lives as they saw fit. In 1961, for instance, before leaving NIMH, he became a founding board member of the National Ballet Society, a position he held until heading up NIA (Brennan & Clarage, 1999:262). Why would a gero-psychiatrist, with children to raise and books to write, spend time promoting dance? He loved ballet, and his wife Diane worked with the company. Besides, Butler was the consummate networker. Boards tend to select people with money, connections, and energy. Washington was a small enough place to reward civic virtue by giving people access to power.

Butler's civic engagement was evident four years later when he founded the Forum for Professionals and Executives in Washington to promote lifelong learning. The forum was modeled after the New York School for Social Research's Institute of Retired Professions (1962). Older learners operated most of the courses and lecture series, which focused on international relations, languages, literature, sciences, and the arts (Boyd & Oakes, 1973:274). As such the initiative must have reminded Butler of what Columbia could offer adult learners. Spin-offs emerged from the forum, which initially had ties with WSP.

In 1969 the Rev. Gregory D. M. Maletta—who later officiated the marriages of Butler and Lewis as well as his daughters Christine and Cynthia—recommended that Butler become involved in an ambitious plan to design a life-care community on a 128-acre preserve close to the Beltway in Prince George's County, Maryland. The site, deeded to the Episcopal Diocese of Washington through the will of William Seton Belt Jr., was to become a "home of aged and retired ministers . . . or for such other charitable purposes of a similar nature" (Bury, 2005). The taskforce expected to tap the talents of retired volunteers with expertise in building codes, health care, and spiritual formation as they created an environment that ran the continuum from independent living to nursing care in a pedestrian-friendly, urban wildlife setting. The project faced opposition from environmentalists, however. Members of the Prince George's County Council feared, moreover, that low-income persons who settled there might require government assistance. The plan was placed on hold.

Butler also offered his services to nonprofit organizations with policy agendas. In 1969, for instance, he joined the board of the National Council on the Aging (NCOA). Smaller and less wealthy than the National Retired Teachers Association—American Association of Retired Persons (now known as AARP), NCOA had an impressive skein of achievements by the time Butler became affiliated with the organization. Its leadership formed the American Association of Homes for the Aged (1961) and, a year later, laid the groundwork for Meals on Wheels. It issued guidelines for Foster Grandparents in 1965. NCOA's sway was critical in persuading Congress to enact the Age Discrimination in Employment Act (1967). The organization negotiated in 1968 the first of many contracts with the Department of Labor to help low-income workers secure employment (Bury, 2005; Pratt, 1967).

Notable persons served on NCOA's board along with Butler. Catherine Dunham, a dancer and anthropologist, sparked his appreciation for Haitian culture, whose art appealed to him and to Myrna Lewis. He interacted with Helen Hayes. He became better acquainted with liberal Republican Arthur Flemming, who offered important mentoring as Butler delved more deeply into policy making for the aged. Flemming and Butler were advisers in the creation of the Fromm Institute of Lifetime Learning in San Francisco. And he formed deep ties with NCOA's newly appointed executive director, Jack Ossofsky, who from 1971 to 1988 would electrify the board with his passion and energy. Support from Flemming and Ossofsky proved critical in securing the NIA director's position for Butler ("Jack Ossofsky," 1992).

Meanwhile, in the wake of the revolution in race relations, Robert Kastenbaum (an iconoclastic psychologist) joined Hobart C. Jackson in convening the National Caucus [and Center] on the Black Caucus (NCBA). Butler was the only other white person besides Kastenbaum on the initial board of trustees. NCBA's immediate concern was that black voices be heard following the 1971 White House Conference on Aging. "There is a lack of awareness of how [the black elderly] are treated in this country," Jackson declared. "They don't understand how racism really works. There is a tendency among black people in general, and especially among older blacks, to accept what we have as being enough" (Achenbaum & Albert, 1995:172; see also Jackson, 1971). NCBA sought to educate members concerning work and health policies, develop housing initiatives to benefit low-income African Americans, and support community-based organizations to assist black elders. (NCBA's aim remains unfulfilled today. For all the current interest in baby boomers on Medicare, the experiences of minority elders, especially African Americans, remains relatively understudied.)

Finally, Butler got policy-making experience in dealing with municipal affairs in the District of Columbia. He held several posts. Initially appointed to the subcommittee on employment for the District of Columbia Interdepartmental Committee on Aging (1966–67), Butler chaired the District of Columbia Advisory Committee on Aging (1969–72). For the District of Columbia Department of Public Health (1970–71), he served on the Mental Health Technical Advisory Committee to the Health Planning Advisory Committee (Brennan & Clarage, 1999:262). These appointments lent credibility to his professional credentials when he offered congressional testimony. And exposure on Capitol Hill, in turn, introduced Butler to kindred spirits advocating for senior citizens at the federal level of government.

"THE PERSONAL IS POLITICAL"

"The personal is political" was an oft-heard feminist rallying cry in the late 1960s and early 1970s. People projected personal crises onto national catastrophes, and vice versa. The slogan seemed terribly relevant to the white middle-class vanguard of the Baby Boom cohort, which had enjoyed considerable advantages while growing up. Suddenly this group found their expectations for a "Great Society" crushed by violence, injustice, and mistrust. Their world seemed to be falling apart before their eyes (Hanisch, 1970; see also Matusow, 1985; O'Neill [1974] 2005).

Boomers were not the only ones affected by the reversal of fortunes transforming the United States. Butler remembered 1968 as a "special year." His outrage over U.S. involvement in Vietnam predated the Tet Offensive early in 1968, he told me. He watched parts of Washington burn after the assassination of Martin Luther King, Jr., in April 1968. Robert Kennedy's murder a few weeks later shocked him. All these events, confided Butler, caused him to reconnect with the pain of poverty, which fanned in turn his anger over racial injustice. His politics and pacifism astounded colleagues and neighbors. Their discomfort and dismay, he assured me, did not deter him from activism.

Although unaffiliated with any faith-based congregation, Butler began to work on issues of race, poverty, and antiwar mobilization with three charismatic clergymen in Washington, Monsignor Geno Baroni, putting Catholic social teaching into action, marched with Dr. King in Selma and served as the Catholic coordinator for the March on Washington for Jobs and Freedom that culminated in King's "I Have a Dream" speech. In 1968 Baroni directed the Urban Task Force of the U.S. Catholic Conference ("The Prominence," 2010; Kirk, 1982:18). As head of the National Presbyterian Church and Center, Philip Newell offered a forum for activists through his center's Woodrow Wilson lectures (Nannes, 1957). The group frequently met at the home of Paul Moore, Jr., who began his ministry in the late 1940s in a predominantly black, inner-city parish in Jersey City; Bishop Moore arguably became the Episcopal Church's best-known representative of the "liberal establishment" ("Episcopal," 2003; Kabaservice, 2004).

Butler was elected from the District of Columbia in 1968 to be an alternate delegate to the National Democratic Convention in Chicago as a supporter of Eugene McCarthy. There he interacted with Arthur Miller and Paul Newman and compared notes with his journalist friend, Bob Maynard, and his daughter Cindy. An eyewitness to the brutalities on Grant Park, Butler identified with the youthful antiwar demonstrators. Although he did not get Bob Dylan's music, he shared their enthusiasm for advancing the cause of love, freedom, and peace.

Never again would Butler's political involvements be so transparent—though for the rest of his life he vigorously supported liberal causes in the face of growing neoconservatism. Butler chose to focus on old-age issues, important in their own right, because (to him) they permeated larger policy challenges. He stressed the interrelatedness of political, economic, social, and physical-mental-psychological health issues embedded in every age-specific problem that he addressed. While he later admitted that he and his contemporaries did not emphasize sufficiently life-course perspectives inherent in geriatrics and gerontology, Butler himself sought to synthesize and convey the evolving big picture.

Butler, understanding that social progress usually took shape in small steps, focused on legislative particulars. He continued to work with Senator Moss and, after 1974, with newly elected congressman David Pryor (the former governor of Arkansas), who endeared himself to Butler by working as a nurse's aide in a District of Columbia facility. In work on legislation on nutrition and the elderly, Butler pooled talents with the legendary Claude Pepper and Sen. Edward M. Kennedy (1975b:269, 289, 330, 41, 196).

Sometimes Robert Butler expressed anger. His frustration is evident over what he considered the modest impact of the 1971 White House Conference on Aging: "Efforts to recognize, define, and measure the problems of the old and to recommend solutions created shelves of reports which are now gathering dust. The 1961 conference, of course, had the excitement of the Medicare fight. But nothing dramatic, compelling, innovative or surprising emerged from the 1971 conference" (Butler, 1975b:331). Butler complained that the conference did too little in addressing the needs of elders with emotional and mental disorders. To move the agenda along during the conference, he nudged a young delegate, Terrie "Fox" Wetle (2010), to speak out on mental-health issues. His disdain for dusty shelves prompted him to keep clippings in folders about cases of old-age discrimination and injustices—materials he would later use while writing *Why Survive?*

Butler's disappointment with the conference did not diminish his esteem for his friend and fellow NCOA board member, Arthur Flemming. "The respected Dr. Arthur S. Flemming, chairman of the White House Conference on Aging, put himself on the line: 'We will speak out in no uncertain terms when action does not keep pace with rhetoric,'" Butler noted. "The politics and the realities of presidential vetoes since the conference have made Flemming's job a difficult one" (Butler, 1975b:334). Butler, like Flemming, realized that more had to be done to raise public consciousness about aging: "The 1960s and '70s saw a crisis of awareness in the United States, increasing the inequities based upon race, sex, class and, to a lesser extent, age. Nineteen-seventy-six marks the two hundredth anniversary of the United States. It also marks another campaign for the presidency. Thus 1976 is an appropriate occasion to press once again the needs of the elderly" (350). Having determined that the nation's bicentennial presented a reasonable deadline for purposive writing, he decided to devote more time to being an author.

BUTLER'S WAY WITH WORDS

Early on, Butler evidently had a gift for coining memorable terms and phrases. "The life review" emerged out of his clinical efforts to guide older clients shaping reminiscences to make sense of the narrative lines of their lives as they neared the end. Half a century later, health-care professionals, gerontologists, and therapists still endorse the concept.

In coining "ageism," Butler (1969) sought to affix a name to a deep and pervasive prejudice, "a form of bigotry we now tend to overlook." Here is his original formulation (1968):

> Ageism can be seen as a process of systematic stereotyping or and discrimination against people because they are old, just as racism and sexism accomplish this with skin color and gender. Old people are categorized as senile, rigid in thought and manner, old-fashioned in morality and skills. Ageism allows the younger generation to see old people as different from themselves; thus they subtly cease to identify with their elders as human beings.
>
> (1975b:12)

From Butler's perspective, ageism operated on individual and institutional planes. He conjectured that disdain and avoidance of aging arose out of ignorance or insufficient contact with elders. People sometimes protected themselves by projecting onto the aged their fear of loss and death. Ageism prevented older Americans from having access to legal, social, transportation, and home-care services. "I first confronted ageism in medical school. We were not taught much about older people, and, indeed, basic knowledge of human aging was minimal," Butler recalled (2005b:xv). "I was shocked by the medical lexicon concerning older persons, abounding as it did with cruel and pejorative terms, such as crock, which was also used to denigrate any woman who was no longer young" (1975b:68–69, 140).

Butler helped to put "ageism" into everyday parlance, frequently using the term (see 1969a:58–60; 1969b:1–9). An article in the *Washington Post* by Carl Bernstein (1969) added visibility. "Ageism" shortly afterward entered the *Oxford English Dictionary.* Scholars and journalists still use the term as Butler formulated it, to describe manifestations of age-based prejudice (see Bytheway 2005; Macnicol 2006; Nelson 2002).

"Ageism plays an important role in the generally negative opinion about mental health care in old age," wrote Butler and Myrna Lewis in the preface to *Aging and Mental Health—Positive Psychosocial Approaches* (1973), which the coauthors declared was the first such comprehensive book on this topic published in the United States. "In this text we hope to dispel some of the traditional diagnostic and treatment myths. We shall be discussing normal healthy aging versus mental illness in old age, age-related problems versus lifelong problems, and endogenous (inside—that is, personality) versus exogenous (outside—that is, environmental) problems" (Butler & Lewis, 1982:xvii–xviii).

Aging and Mental Health "aimed for a down-to-earth, practical approach . . . while at the same time introducing the basic terminology of the field" (xix). The pair split assignments. Lewis contributed the notion of "responsible dependency" as an adaptive mode utilized by healthy elders substituting satisfactions for losses; Butler wrote about pharmacology.

The book has two sections. Part 1 offers a profile of healthy successful aging and surveys common emotional problems and various functional and organic disorders. "In providing information about old age, we do not espouse fields such as geriatric psychiatry, geriatric psychology, and geriatric social work," Butler and Lewis asserted. "This information should be part of a core therapy of the life cycle of human beings rather than a separate entity" (xviii). Based on new insights into caring for older persons, part 2 highlights active interventions and possibilities for restorative, rehabilitative treatment. "Older people need a *restitution capacity*, the ability to compensate for and recover from deeply losses," the authors stressed. "They also need the opportunity for *growth and renewal*" (193–94).

Aging and Mental Health fit a niche with therapists and clinicians, who praised its scope, eclectic perspective, and standardized clinical forms and lexicons of bureaucratic terms (Berkman, 1978:230–45; Liebig, 1983:124–32; Mensh, 1974:405). The authors suffused the book with vignettes and photographs, attesting to the diversity of older Americans, as they wrestled with policy issues left unresolved after the 1971 White House Conference on Aging. A revised version appeared in 1977, and the book eventually went through five editions.

In several respects, *Why Survive? Being Old in America* (1975) resembles *Aging and Mental Health*. They are big books—nearly five hundred pages in length—crammed with statistics and citations. Encyclopedic in scope, both works seek to alter the thinking of professionals and a reading public. Butler expressed a hope that "this book informs, illuminates, angers and guides its readers" (1975b:x). By making the rage behind many of his words explicit at the outset, Butler forewarned his audience: *Why Survive?* is a jeremiad that deploys rational thinking and civil discourse to propose a radical shift in attitudes toward age and aging, particularly in the policy arena.

Butler issued statements at several times over his career about what prompted him to write *Why Survive?* His series of commentaries offer consistent glimpses into his thoughts and feelings. In his 1975 blurb "About the Author," he claimed that "his activities over the past twenty years encompass research and observation, clinical practice, writing, muckraking and public advocacy" (1975b:498). These varied experiences and long-standing engagement as an advocate for older Americans, he affirmed, entitled him to represent himself as a seasoned participant-observer who desired to redirect the hearts and minds of professional colleagues and fellow citizens. Also helpful were the $30,000 advance, which freed six months for writing; cogent advice from Ann Harris, his "superb editor" who urged him to reduce the text by a third; and Myrna Lewis's editorial assistance.

Two decades later Butler proudly claimed that *Why Survive?* was a catalyst for new U.S. old-age policies and that simultaneously spurred fresh ways of re-presenting late life:

> This work provided a portrait of old age in America and offered policy solutions. It included a critique of deinstitutionalization, the commercial nursing home industry, medicine, psychiatry, and other professional fields in meeting the needs of older persons. It encouraged passage of the Age Discrimination in Employment Act and the end of mandatory retirement. *Why Survive?* was the stimulus for the Pulitzer-prize winning play, *The Gin Game.*
>
> (ACHENBAUM & ALBERT, 1995:64)

Thirty years later after its publication, Butler declared that *Why Survive?* "presented an indictment of ageism in American society and suggested ideas for comprehensive reforms" (2005b:xv). And with this utterance, the author came full circle.

Putting the finishing touches on *Why Survive?*, Butler wrote late in 1974, pushed him into unfamiliar territory: "In my own twenty years of work with older people as a physician, researcher, psychiatrist, and participant in community and public affairs, I have been forced to go beyond the traditional confines of medicine to look at cultural attitudes and economic circumstances." Connections made in Washington, intellectual, clinical, social, and political, had prepared Robert Butler, then in his late forties, to ask himself and his audience a fundamental question: were Americans individually or collectively willing to settle for "mere survival" in later years? "As this book went to press in early 1975, the situation of the average older American was becoming increasingly desperate" (1975b:xiii). There was no time to waste, in his opinion. Here was a social problem potentially as significant as racism and sexism.

"Old age is often a tragedy"—those were Butler's first words in his preface. "Few of us like to consider it because it reminds of us our own mortality" (xi). While the rest of the paragraph reminded readers of their fears of deformity and death, and their dreaded association of aging with dying, Butler did not intend to write a sequel to Ernest Becker's *Denial of Death*, which had won the Pulitzer Prize in 1974. Butler wrote *Why Survive?* to document and excoriate the impoverishment of late life in America. He wanted in plain language to expose the unnecessary, often unwitting, hardships that millions of older people endured before they experienced death.

Butler was appalled by a scourge that stripped meaning and dignity from virtually every aspect of life for vulnerable segments of the elderly population. A keyword in *Why Survive?* was *tragedy*. "For many elderly Americans old age is a tragedy, a period of quiet despair, desperation, desolation, and muted rage. . . . We have shaped a society which is extremely harsh to live in when one is old. The tragedy of old age is not the fact that each of us must grow old and die but that the process of doing so has been made unnecessarily and at times excruciatingly painful, humiliating, debilitating and isolating through insensitivity, ignorance and poverty" (2–3).

In retrospect, it seems ironic that *Why Survive?* focused so much on old age's tragic features. After all, contemporary gerontologists—Butler's peers—were stressing age's positive features, such as the capacities of elders to adapt and adjust. To stir imaginations, however, Butler decided to accentuate the problems.

Why Survive? thus fleshed out a problem-oriented agenda. The first eight chapters followed one another thematically, dealing with economics and work; housing and home-health services; drugs and substance abuse; and emotional problems and mental illness. The next two revisited nursing-home scandals and victimization of older people. They were followed by a pair of chapters on the politics of aging and a policy agenda for what Butler described as the "gift of life." In the penultimate chapter he addressed marriage and education in order to propose ways of breaking out of age-based institutional arrangements. Chapter 14, entitled "Growing Up Absurd," highlighted life review's value in counseling.

Butler did not borrow the organization that he and Lewis laid out in *Aging and Mental Health.* Chapters in *Why Survive?* function as self-contained units; there is no red thread through successive chapters culminating in a story line to a grand conclusion. That the chapters and consultants were compartmentalized reflects how he organized clippings and citations in separate folders. Yet Butler's portrayal of "A More Balanced View of Old Age" (408), which emphasized the heterogeneity of elderly persons, was one place that he told readers what healthy aging may promise if ageism diminished, living conditions improved, and the needs of older people were given a higher priority in U.S. policy-making circles.

Butler was forty-nine when he received the 1976 Pulitzer Prize for General Non-Fiction and glowing reviews. He was the first—and thus far, the only—geriatrician and gerontologist so honored. Norman Cousins, one of the judges, became a close friend several years after the prize was announced. Other colleagues, such as Judd Marmor in the *New York Times Book Review,* saluted Butler's achievement as "important, fact-filled, compassionate, and insightful." Alex Comfort, MD, pronounced it "the best and best informed exposé to appear so far . . . every American of every age should read this book"—an endorsement seconded by the American Medical Association" (Amazon.com).

The central message of *Why Survive?* survives for a new generation of readers to absorb. Butler plainly demonstrated that it takes more than a multidisciplinary, life-course perspective to peel away the myths and stereotypes of being old. People need some grounding in basic science, social relations, and modern-day political economies—not to mention an appreciation for the varieties of policy making that transpired in households, within institutional residences, and in statehouses and the Capitol—to understand the diverse needs of America's heterogeneous old-age population, which was rapidly increasing in size. At a more basic level, Butler insisted, people had to appreciate the contrarieties of growing older, its assets and uncertainties. Looking seriously at the challenges and opportunities presented in late life, urged *Why Survive?*, required individual of all ages to look backward and forward both to old age's intrinsic meanings and to the ways that individual choices and societal expectations converge in the web of policy making.

❧ ❧ ❧ ❧ ❧

Two other fundamental transitions in Butler's life between 1963 and 1975 merit note. By ending this chapter this way, I mean to highlight their significance, not to present these events as an afterthought. The dissolution and subsequent formation of two intimate bonds deeply affected Butler's thoughts, emotions, and behavior. His marriage to Diane McLaughlin unraveled; she asked him for a divorce in 1971. Eschewing the usual pattern of midlife male behavior, Butler chose not to remarry quickly. He wanted to give his daughters (Chris, Carole, and Cindy)—to whom he dedicated *Why Survive?*—a chance to adjust to this change. He, too, needed time to come to terms with the ramifications of the breakup for his family life. Hence Robert Butler and Myrna Lewis waited until 1975 to wed. His esteemed co-therapist and coauthor, despite their differences, became the great love of Butler's life.

five
BUTLER AT THE NATIONAL INSTITUTE ON AGING

Interviewing Butler in 1976, shortly after he assumed responsibilities at the National Institute on Aging (NIA), an official from the American Hospital Association characterized the founding director as "militant and mild, aggressive and compassionate; he is the ideal physician-scientist to take on the heavy responsibilities that confront elderly Americans" (Lesparre, 1976:50). To his new post Butler brought vision, energy, passion, tact, and survival instincts. Over the next six years he would deploy skills and stratagems that he had refined as a scientist, psychiatrist, and advocate. He knew how to communicate to powerbrokers in Washington, D.C., as well as to lay constituencies fervently and persuasively about the importance of research to improve the health and well-being of older Americans.

From the start NIA's future success was uncertain. Formidable foes inside the National Institutes of Health (NIH) and the executive branch, not to mention research communities across the nation, opposed P.L. 93–296, the Research on Aging Act (1974), which authorized NIH's eleventh institute. It had an amorphous mandate and diffuse constituency. Although President Ford's appointment of Butler to be NIA's first director got through

Congress, he was not the obvious frontrunner for the post. Money was tight at all institutes on the Bethesda campus; NIA's initial budget was modest.

In short order Butler needed to articulate a strategic action plan at once sensible, feasible, and compelling. He had to generate and mobilize support for NIA among leaders on Capitol Hill, in medical schools and major academic centers, and in the media. Butler had to persuade diverse audiences that the pay-offs from basic and applied research on aging could relieve suffering and promote healthfulness in later years—and do so as effectively as science and technology had done in curing childhood illnesses and advancing public health.

RELUCTANTLY EXPANDING RESEARCH ON AGING

Virtually every health economist in the 1970s concurred that biomedical research had reduced mortality rates and the costs of disease in the United States during the twentieth century. Scientific advances accounted for roughly 40 percent of the reductions in "objective sickness." Research investments lowered costs associated with premature deaths and illness (Mushkin, 1979). NIH unquestionably had played a major role in this success story.

"The National Institutes of Health is not only the largest institution for biomedical science on earth, it is one of this nation's great treasures," declared Dr. Lewis Thomas, president emeritus of New York's Memorial Sloan-Kettering Medical Center. "As social inventions for human betterment go, this one is a standing proof that, at least once in a while, government possesses the capacity to do something unique, imaginative, and altogether right." Noting that intramural research represented only 10 percent of NIH's budget, Thomas added that "for sheer excellence and abundant productivity the institution cannot be matched by any other scientific enterprise anywhere." Roughly 2,220 of the 14,000 staff on the Bethesda campus had doctorates, half of them MDs, and six were Nobel laureates. Forty-five investigators produced a sixth of the 300 most cited articles in the biosciences (Stetten & Carrigan, 1984:4).

Research on aging had not kept pace with scientific advances at NIH or elsewhere, however. In 1940 Surgeon General Thomas Parran and National Institutes of Health director Lewis R. Thompson expressed interest in studying "degenerative disorders" associated with geriatrics in order to encourage research into chronic diseases. With support from the Josiah Macy Jr. Foundation, the U.S. Public Health Service asked Edward Stieglitz to survey current research on aging. In addition NIH formed a freestanding research unit to (1) map out biological processes of senescence and (2) study "the human clinical problems of aging and of diseases characteristically associated with advancing years" (Lockett, 1983:32). Nathan W. Shock, a Berkeley physiologist, was recruited in 1941 to head a gerontological lab established in the Baltimore City Hospitals (BCH). The outbreak of World War II suspended operations, but in 1948 BCH provided a fortybed ward devoted exclusively to the Section on Gerontology. Shock remained a key figure in developing NIH's research agenda on aging until he died in 1989.

Nathan Shock and the Section on Gerontology were not the only federal agents supporting research on aging in postwar America. The National Institute on Mental Health, as we have seen, underwrote two volumes of *Human Aging*. Findings issued by the National Cancer Institute often proved pertinent to work being undertaken by gerontologists and geriatricians. Meanwhile Dr. James Watt, who headed the National Heart Institute from 1952 to 1961, promoted extramural research on aging. When a Gerontology Study Section at NIH dissolved because of the paucity and mediocrity of proposals for funding it received compared to other review panels, Congress allocated funds in 1956 to create a Center on Aging Research at NIH and multidisciplinary centers for aging research and training in medical schools at Brown, Duke, Case Western, University of Miami, and Albert Einstein in New York's Yeshiva University. Only Duke's center flourished. Lackluster results once again disappointed advocates and, more importantly, solidified resistance among those who did not much want NIH to become more involved in aging research (Lockett, 1983:34–42).

One major opponent was Dr. James A. Shannon, NIH director from 1955 to 1968, who doubled the number of personnel and launched three institutes, thanks to sound intellectual values and good managerial decisions (Kennedy, 1994; Shannon, 1971). Consistent with Shannon's *festina lento* approach to budgetary details was his refusal to dilute standards or diffuse NIH's focus. "At any level of federal expenditure for health," Shannon declared, "the distribution of support among the related activities subtended, and the terms and conditions of the support, are at least as important as the absolute levels of support which obtain" (Shannon, 1974:3311). Since it was hard to cultivate common values and to sustain productivity within various institutes, Shannon urged Congress not to burden NIH's mission by adding new priorities.

Three institutes—Mental Health, Child Health and Human Development, and Cancer—underwrote research on aging before NIA. Their histories underscore the intellectual and strategic balance that Shannon sought to maintain between seeking short-term scientific advantages and nurturing long-term benefits. These institutes offered insights into the contested NIH values and politics that Butler knew he would face at the National Institute on Aging.

The National Institute of Mental Health was established in 1949 to address turf wars between social scientists and biomedical researchers and analytic versus clinical approaches to diseases such as schizophrenia amid profound changes in psychoanalytic theories and behavioral practices. "Of all the Institutes brought together to constitute the National Institutes of Health, the National Institute of Mental Health was the least firmly based on an accepted foundation of rigorous scientific research" (Stetten & Carrigan, 1984:13). When the Kennedy administration wanted to fight mental retardation, its request fomented discord among NIMH, psychiatrists in private practice, and the American Association on Mental Deficiency. Notwithstanding myriad tensions, NIMH was considered a successful research incubator and training center. Alcohol and substance abuse were added to its purview in the late 1960s and early 1970s; in 1975 gero-psychiatrist Gene D. Cohen, MD, PhD, took charge of NIMH's Center on Aging, the first such government-funded unit in the world (Achenbaum, 2010).

If NIMH's history illustrated stakeholder truculence in defining mental illness and promoting mental health in a multidisciplinary research setting, the establishment of the National Institute of Child Health and Human Development (NICHD) revealed other scientific fissures that had political consequences. President Kennedy wanted to give priority to the health needs of young Americans despite resistance from legal counsel and Abraham Ribicoff, his secretary of Health, Education, and Welfare (HEW). Shannon noted that the Institutes of Neurology, Heart, and Cancer already were addressing children's issues. Also at stake was the role to be played by social or behavioral scientists and clinicians. Nonetheless Kennedy moved ahead, and Congress authorized the creation of the new institute in 1962. NIH accepted its inevitability, "asking for as much as we can get out of it in exchange for adopting the little waif" (Lockett, 1983:59–61). Kennedy's men, members of Congress, NIH administrators, and outside experts paid little attention to how research on aging might develop within the proposed institute. They ignored a recommendation from the 1961 White House Conference on Aging that NIH should establish an Institute of Gerontology.

Finally, the successful expansion of the National Cancer Institute, NIH's first categorical disease institute, showed Butler the importance of philanthropic activists. More than $2 billion had been appropriated to NCI, established in 1937; by 1970 its annual budget approached $200 million, an outlay many deemed insufficient to the task. "Our government this year spent, per person in the United States, $410 on national defense, $19 on foreign aid and $125 on the Indochina War," observed Sen. Ralph W. Yarborough (D-TX) in 1970. "In the vital field of cancer research—to study a disease that will kill 330,000 of our people in one year—this government spent only 89 cents per person" (Rettig, 1977:1, 8).

Determined to redirect dollars for cancer research on a scale analogous to a "Moon Shot," Senator Yarborough worked closely with philanthropist Mary Lasker, who, with Florence Mahoney, raised federal appropriations for biomedical research during the 1950s and 1960s. Lasker's citizen lobby collaborated with top NIH administrators and congressional leaders in securing passage of the 1971 National Cancer Act (P.L. 92–218). The landmark measure, however, often put scientists' research aims at odds with the managerial priorities of lawmakers and scientific administrators, among other stakeholders, as well as private citizens appointed to advisory boards. Shannon opined that "scientific judgments frequently got lost in, or unnecessarily and improperly diluted" (Rettig, 1977:138–39, 150).

The National Cancer Act raised hitherto unspoken, possibly overlooked questions about aspects of NIH's mission. Would all institutes be expected to privilege pathways that promised to conquer disease? How should experts valorize efforts to understand processes that promote healthful living? How far ought popular opinions about disease risks be taken into account? What balance, fiscal and intellectual, should exist between generating basic research and applying new knowledge?

Such questions would never be resolved, of course, but in the debates research on aging received short shrift for two reasons. First, there were insufficient numbers of credible researchers in the aging field. Second, NIH's leadership plausibly claimed that an infrastructure already existed to promote gerontology. Forces nonetheless converged in the early 1970s that made it possible for advocates to establish an institute on aging on NIH's campus.

Delegates to the 1971 White House Conference on Aging recommended that "a National Institute of Gerontology be established immediately to support and conduct research and training in the bio-medical and social-behavioral aspects of aging" (U.S. Senate 1971:47). The Gerontological Society, the National Council on Aging, and the National Council of Senior Citizens backed the proposal. The National Retired Teachers Association—American Association of Retired Persons, one of the nation's largest and fastest-growing organizations, representing nearly three million members, also endorsed the idea (Pratt, 1976; Walker, 1991).

An NIH-based aging institute had support from well-placed lobbyists and congressional leaders. Florence Mahoney, Mary Lasker's comrade in arms who had been active in Washington circles since the Truman era, made this cause her top priority. Mahoney had raised funds for NIH research on arthritis and heart disease. Unlike Lasker, who thought that breakthroughs in cancer and heart research would fully solve major problems in aging, Mahoney wanted to concentrate on improving the quality of older Americans' lives and fighting the ravages of dementia.

In 1972 Florence Mahoney enlisted help from Rep. Paul G. Rogers (D-FL), "Mr. Health" in Congress. When Senator Yarborough proved lukewarm in his commitment, she turned to Sen. Tom Eagleton (D-MO), who chaired a Senate committee on aging (Baranaukus, 2002; Hevesi, 2008; Robinson, 2001). With fourteen important cosponsors, Senator Eagleton called for the creation of a National Institute of Gerontology, quickly followed by a proposal by Senator Harrison Williams (D-NJ) for the Research on Aging Act.

There were obstacles. Richard Nixon, wishing to contain expenses, vetoed measures to establish an institute; he was too ensnared after 1973 in Watergate to much care, however. HEW officials resisted creating another institute. A new cohort of NIH leaders joined the American Association of Medical Colleges in opposition (Lockett, 1983:92, 122, 132–33).

Internal disagreements within the nascent gray lobby almost derailed the coalition. Some advocates wanted a disease focus, while others stressed multidisciplinary and applied research into mechanisms and processes of growing older. Lewis Thomas's opinion (1972:16)—"If I were a policymaker, interested in saving money over the long haul, I would regard it as an act of prudence to give high priority to a lot more basic research in biological sciences"—prevailed. Florence Mahoney, sharing the view of several prominent bio-gerontologists, did not want social scientists and behaviorists in the proposed institute. Others preferred that the Administration on Aging or some other federal agency besides NIH oversee research activities and budget requests in this area.

Richard Nixon in 1974 signed Public Law 93-296, establishing the National Institute on Aging under NIH "for the conduct and support of biomedical, social, and behavioral research and training related to the aging process and the diseases and other special problems and needs of the aged." The first task was to establish, in consultation with the HEW secretary and a duly appointed National Advisory Council on Aging, the foci of "research in the biological, medical, psychological, social, educational and economic aspects of aging" (sect. 464). The law also required translating research not just to scientific and academic communities but to citizen consumers: "The Institute shall carry out public information and education programs designed to disseminate as widely as possible the findings of Institute-sponsored and other relevant aging research and studies and other information about the processes of aging which may assist elderly and near-elderly persons in dealing with, and all Americans in understanding, the problems and processes associated with growing older" (sect. 463[c]).

Finding a suitable director for NIA came next. Several likely candidates did not wish to give up the salaries and security they enjoyed in academic settings. Stanford University microbiologist Leonard Hayflick became a prime contender (Hayflick & Moorhead, 1961). Hayflick's NIA candidacy was undermined, however, by a six-year lawsuit settled out of court concerning whether he owned and could sell cell tissues that he had cultured under an NIH grant (Achenbaum & Albert, 1995:162). When no obvious biomedical scientist emerged as a top candidate, other people's names surfaced as possibilities. After reading *Why Survive?* Florence Mahoney recommended Butler, whom she found "absolutely sensational." Mahoney, with strong support from Arthur Flemming, Eisenhower's HEW secretary who had chaired the 1971 White House Conference on Aging, contacted Dr. Theodore Cooper at HEW; Dr. Donald Frederickson, the new NIH director; and Dr. Ronald Lamont-Havers, the NIH deputy director who chaired the search committee. Butler told me that he met once with the search committee (which included Nathan Shock) and recalled having two conversations, largely philosophical, with Frederickson (National Library; Butler, personal communication, January 2, 2010). He impressed everyone.

Speaking before the American Geriatrics Society days before becoming founding director of the National Institute on Aging, Butler could hardly contain his excitement. "I feel as if I have been given a midlife research career development award with an incredible opportunity to try to do something constructive toward shaping research and training in America," he declared. Butler did not underestimate the challenges. "This institute is going to need all of your ideas and support in order to grow in an orderly, progressive and sensible fashion (Butler, 2003b).

DEVELOPING A RESEARCH AND TRAINING PLAN
AT NIA FOR *OUR FUTURE SELVES*

From the outset, Butler told me, he and Frederickson had an understanding unlike the norm for NIH directors. Butler could move freely on Capitol

Hill as long as he did not embarrass his boss or the institutes. In return, Frederickson promised to leave the new NIA director alone (Butler, personal communication, January 2, 2010). The arrangement did not always work to Butler's advantage: when budget requests were due, Frederickson rarely went out of his way to help NIA since he presumed that Butler appeared quite capable of taking care of himself.

Butler proudly related to me that he altered another protocol. Institute directors usually did not interact with one another except in scheduled meetings with the NIH director. Butler made it a point to walk across the Bethesda campus and introduce himself to each of his new colleagues. His overture facilitated subsequent efforts to initiate collaborative ventures.

Having studied the history of NIH and its institutes and divisions (Butler, 1976), Butler clearly understood that NIA's mandate was statutorily different from those of other institutes—its multidisciplinary thrust focused on neither organ nor disease. To grow a credible and viable institute, he had to make sure its research met NIH's highest standards. However he enunciated objectives, he faced skepticism. Misconceptions about the aims and outcomes of aging research were rampant. Butler at every turn confronted ageism and fallacies about senescence. Accordingly, he consistently argued that research could generate effective social and medical old-age interventions only by disentangling intrinsic and extrinsic changes associated with senescence (NIA, 1978).

Besides correcting blind spots about aging, there were other challenges. Tight money made choices tough. In fiscal year 1975 HEW spent $25–30 million on research directly related to older people. NIA's initial budget was only $19.3 million, or 1 percent of NIH's research budget (Fox, 1989:96; NIA, 1977:56). But NIA's capacities were limited by more than fiscal constraints. Butler tactfully saluted research on aging done by other HEW agencies as he deflected dubious proposals or requests forwarded to his desk because they had "age" in their subject heading (Butler, 2003b:1170; NIA, 1978:54–55). Faced with doubts about aging research, Butler could not sound overly confident about possibilities for curing diseases and ameliorating disabilities. At the same time he had to dispel that sense of nihilism or fatalism about late-life decline and loss that had long bedeviled the field (Achenbaum, 1978; Butler, 1976:294).

In late 1976 NIA issued *Our Future Selves: A Research Plan Toward Understanding Aging.* Not only was the title inspired, but the plan underscored the stake that citizens of all ages had in confronting distortions about aging: "The distortion is imposed by two elements: the vital supports which many of the elderly lose merely by the fact of having become aged; and our ignorance of what aging is—an ignorance made the more profound by our societal resistance to acknowledging the fact of aging and preparing adequately for it" (NIA, 1977:1). The blueprint was designed to have widespread appeal. It showcased the power of multidisciplinary connectedness that gerontologists valued. (In retrospect, Butler admitted that the agenda was so ambitious that it overwhelmed people.) In consultation with the National Advisory Council on Aging, *Our Future Selves* listed ten short-term and long-term "selected research opportunities" for each of three aging-related research areas mandated by Congress:

- Under biomedical issues, it included studies of diseases common to the aged, to be studied in collaboration with other NIH institutes and HEW agencies.
- Under behavioral/social issues, it included improvement and maintenance of memory.
- Under issues in human services and delivery was the cost of elder care. "If we can find better ways to deliver health care to the aged, the lessons learned may be applied to the delivery of effective and economic health care to the society-at-large" (14).

For the rest of his career, Robert Butler emphasized the importance of basic research on aging along the lines he enunciated at NIA. Training specialists in aging, in his opinion, would augment research resources. "Gerontology and longevity science are surely magnet fields of the 21st century," he wrote. "Underlying all of this planning is the realization that the ultimate health-care service and, indeed, the ultimate health-care cost containment mechanisms result from fundamental research. Research is much less expensive than dealing after the fact with growing numbers of diseased and disabled elderly people" (Butler, 1993a).

ALZHEIMER'S DISEASE AS A RESEARCH PRIORITY

From the beginning of his tenure, Butler understood that scientists and government officials were not NIA's only stakeholders. "The public does not see itself as 'suffering' from the basic biology of aging, nor does it generally believe that aging per se can be reversed. Rather the public has come to view medical research as contributing to an understanding of specific diseases associated with old age" (Butler, 1999:389–90). He needed to showcase a disease to mobilize grassroots support. "We had to put Alzheimer's on the map," he recalled, seizing on senility. "It's much more common than was suspected in those days" (Kastor, 2010:93).

Butler's choice of Alzheimer's, hardly a household word in the 1970s, was not accidental. He had experience dealing with the disease. He had studied dementia as well as healthy aging at NIMH. He had observed patients at St. Elizabeth's Hospital and discussed their tangles and plaques with its neuropathologist, Meta Newman. Dr. Leroy Duncan, who then spearheaded NICHD's extramural program, wanted dementia to be a priority at NIA. Yet Alzheimer's had attracted little interest in scientific communities. Butler in 1975 identified only a dozen grants on it sponsored by NIH.

Alzheimer's disease was worth pursuing, Butler thought, because it would give NIA visibility in scientific communities and the public square. "Success frequently derived from what I came to call the 'health politics of anguish,' that is, public concern about a specific disease, expressed by families who have suffered and by advocacy groups" (Butler, 1999:389; Shabahangi, 2009). Although "the health politics of anguish" touched a nerve, Butler made Alzheimer's a priority when NIA had little money or credibility. Few psychiatrists and psychologists were interested in the disease. There was nothing comparable to the American Cancer Society advocating for Alzheimer's. No one could raise money like the March of Dimes (Oshinsky, 2005:188). Butler nonetheless figured that dementia would become a major health issue as the Baby Boom cohort reached advanced ages. Sharing this opinion was Lewis Thomas, who in 1981 christened Alzheimer's "the disease of the century" (Butler, 1996:xiii; Thomas, 1983:121; see also Levine, 2004).

Several developments quickly came together. First, partly in response to an appeal by Dr. Robert Katzman, who projected startling future increases in cases of Alzheimer's disease, Butler (in collaboration with the directors of NIMH and the National Institute of Neurological and Communicative Disorders and Stroke [NINCDS]) decided to sponsor a symposium in 1977 on "Alzheimer's Disease—Senile Dementia and Related Disorders." The proceedings became the benchmark for evaluating research options concerning the causes and prevalence of the diseases and proposals for new treatment approaches. "The problems are important," NINCDS director Donald Tower opined. "The challenges are extraordinary." Butler agreed:

> Aging is characterized by alterations in the major human integrative systems, such as the immune and central nervous systems. These changes may leave the body vulnerable to disease, but disease is not the inevitable outcome of aging. . . . It is only through research that we can obtain the necessary new knowledge that will lead to prevention of the diseases of old age. Research thus can be viewed as the ultimate service, the ultimate cost-container.
>
> (1982:6; SEE ALSO BALLENGER, 2006; FOX 1999;
> KATZMAN, TERRY, & BICK, 1978)

Second, Butler hired Zaven Khachaturian in 1978 to head a Neurobiology of Aging program, which initially focused on biocognitive changes associated with normal aging and then was to shepherd competitive projects on Alzheimer's disease through the review process. To complement Khachaturian's efforts, Butler created a Laboratory of Neurosciences, added a Section on Stress and Coping in the Gerontology Research Center in Baltimore, and expanded initiatives for extramural research by developing a Neurology Section as part of NIA's Geriatrics Branch and a Basic Neurology Section as part of its Physiology of Aging Branch. He also stimulated work on Alzheimer's disease sponsored through NIA collaborations with NIMH, NINCDS, the National Institute of Allergy and Infectious Diseases, and the National Institute of Occupational Safety and Health (Butler, 1982; Fox, 1989).

The National Institute on Aging benefited from these initiatives. The *Journal of the American Medical Association* issued a task force report on "Senility Reconsidered" in 1980, which included a form with which to evaluate a patient's mental status (NIA, 1980). And NIA profited, though not as much as Butler hoped. Funding for research on Alzheimer's disease increased from $2.3 million to $4.3 million between 1976 and 1980.

Giving priority to Alzheimer's yielded another dividend. Dr. Butler helped to organize a citizen's lobby, modeled after the American Heart Association, to raise consciousness and money to fight dementia. There were a dozen groups in the United States and Canada independently interested in Alzheimer's. So he teamed with Robert Katzman (who had obtained tax-exempt status for an Alzheimer's Disease Society in New York), Florence Mahoney, and Donald Tower in bringing together interested parties to try to coordinate efforts.

Central to the initiative was Jerome Stone, a prominent businessman whose wife was afflicted with the disease. In 1980 Stone became chair of the new, nonprofit Alzheimer's Disease and Related Disorder's Association (ADRDA), which formed a Public Policy and Advocacy Committee as well as a Medical and Scientific Advisory Board (Ballenger, 2006:116–18). Princess Yasmin Aga Khan, whose mother Rita Hayworth had Alzheimer's, joined the board. "Dear Abby" made readers aware of people's pain when she published a letter from "Desperate in New York" under the headline "Memory Disease Can't Be Forgotten." Through links made by NIA's public information office, ADRDA received nearly forty thousand responses to this column alone (Fox, 1989:86; Johnson, 2010; Khan, n.d.).

Media attention paid off. "Around here Congress tends to pay more attention to popular media than scientific journals," Khachaturian observed (Fox, 1989:89). By 1981, when successful Alzheimer's-related proposals accounted for 41 percent of NIA's extramural funding, Congress raised allocations for NIA.

Not everybody was happy. A few critics suggested that NIA be renamed the National Institute on Alzheimer's. Some biologists derided "the Alzheimerization of Aging," asserting that funds for the study and treatment of disease were disproportionate to resources available to pursue other priorities (Adelman, 1995; Butler, 1999; see also Gilman & Foster, 1996). Peter J. Whitehouse, a world-class Alzheimer's expert who lauded Butler's efforts to garner media attention to aging research through the aegis of "the health politics of anguish," was troubled in a different way: "Nuance was lost, sacrificed on the altar of political expediency," he noted. "Few were willing to tell the AD emperors that their vestments were a bit more transparent than they thought" (Whitehouse & George, 2008:96).

Rather than respond directly in print to Whitehouse's concerns, Butler stressed a more general point: "We can all learn from the AIDS, breast cancer, and Alzheimer's disease movements to be forceful advocates" (1999:391). In an era of tight funds and short attention spans, Butler believed, advancing research required allies outside the labs. Taking the "anguish" of Alzheimer's to heart, he argued, opened paths to Big Science: "We need an aggressive national program in Alzheimer's disease, part of an aggressive national program of gerontology and geriatric medicine, a program that is itself part of an advancing frontier in basic research" (Butler, 1982:387).

To meet NIA's mandate, basic research at the institute could not be limited to bench science and clinical medicine. Butler wanted to establish an interdisciplinary program. That meant recruiting broadly to attract the best talent available. Whereas many NIH directors were wary of recruiting behavioral and social scientists, Butler welcomed those who did rigorous work. After sociologist Glen Elder (who wrote the *Children of the Great Depression*) turned him down, Butler enlisted James Birren to help him recruit Matilda White Riley, whose three-volume *Aging and Society* (1968–71) distinguished between works in gerontology that contributed to science and those that did not. Riley in turn recruited Marcia Ory and Richard Suzman, who augmented NIA's intramural strengths and supported significant extramural research on aging.

Multidisciplinary work in gerontology, Butler decided, required greater buttresses. This explains his decision to develop richer longitudinal data banks on aging. For instance, the Framington Heart Study (2010), beginning with 5,200 men and women between ages thirty and sixty-two in 1948 and adding another 5,100 of their children and spouses in 1971, proved indispensable in identifying patterns related to cardiovascular disease. He was also impressed by Ralph Paffenbarger's analysis of the risk of death due to sedentary and vigorous lifestyles among 17,000 Harvard graduates ranging between ages thirty and eighty (Pearce, 2007).

NIA developed its own longitudinal baseline. In 1958 Nathan Shock recruited 1,000 male volunteers between the ages of seventeen and ninety-six for the Baltimore Longitudinal Study of Aging (BLSA), which distinguished normal physical and mental mechanisms and processes of aging from disease, socioeconomic deprivation, and educational disadvantage. Butler insisted that women be added to the study; the BLSA Women's Program began in 1978. NIA also added a Stress and Coping Section to BLSA to measure how subjects adapted to life changes.

Butler also established an Epidemiology, Demography, and Biometry Program (EDBP) to explore the relationship between economic status and health while it probed connections among family structure, physical environment, and health. He tapped Dr. Jacob Brody, a prominent epidemiologist who had worked at the Centers for Disease Control and designed an alcoholism and drug abuse study at the National Institute of Alcohol Abuse and Alcoholism, to head the venture (Brody, Cornoni-Huntley, & Patrick, 1981; Stayner, 2008). EDBP under Brody reported that age-related diseases increased logarithmically; without effective preventive measures, years were added to life without adding health to life. Brody built networks at Harvard, Yale, Iowa, Duke, and the University of Texas Medical Branch at Galveston, and he provided training funds for junior investigators such as Lisa Berkman and Adrian Ostfeld.

In response to outcry over the Tuskegee syphilis scandal (1971), Butler and his staff complied with new federal ethical standards. Sometimes they found that enforcing ethical guidelines with human subjects affected

initiatives at NIA. He told me that ethical issues stymied his efforts to recruit more older people in clinical drug tests. They also served to deter
Butler from adding biomarkers to his research agenda. Chronological age
predicted little of importance to senescence, he knew, but scientists recognized that caloric reduction in rats typically extended longevity. Designing
suitable biomarkers in aging might have refined measurements and predic-
tions about the rate at which organisms age (Baker & Sprott, 1998; Miller,
2001; Turturro et al., 1999). Still, critics worried that ill-conceived biomarkers might cause harm by reducing the autonomy of women and men
in laboratory settings. Problems in disentangling late-life changes and the
onset of diseases, phenomena occurring simultaneously in cells and multiple organs in humans and other mammals, moreover, complicated the creation of biomarkers.

TRAINING HEALTH-CARE PROFESSIONALS TO MEET THE NEEDS OF AN AGING POPULATION

P.L. 93-296, the Research on Aging Act, declared that the HEW "secretary may also provide training and instruction and establish traineeships
and fellowships, in [NIA] and elsewhere, in matters relating to study and
investigation of the aging process and the diseases and other special needs
of the aged." The act also stipulated that "adequate numbers of allied
health nursing and paramedical personnel in the field of health care for the
aged" be trained (sect. 463[a][2]). There was an acute shortage of general
practitioners and specialists versed in geriatrics. "There were no trained
geriatricians; no geriatrics faculty to develop model geriatrics care programs, train geriatricians, educate medical students, residents, or practicing physicians, or conduct aging-related research," William R. Hazzard
recalled (2004:289–303).

To discern how best to proceed, Butler asked David Hamburg, head of
the Institute of Medicine (IoM) at the National Academy of Sciences, to
identify content areas and assess effective teaching methods. Dr. Hamburg
in turn enlisted Dr. Paul Beeson, who regretted "the relative neglect" of
geriatric teaching and practice in the United States compared to England

(Yoshikawa, 2006a, 2006b). Having spent his career in academic settings involved in acute medicine and tertiary care, Beeson initially reckoned that faculty in departments of medicine knew plenty about geriatrics. He soon realized that he himself had much to learn about being old. Many caregivers were ageist, indifferent to the long-term needs of their older patients.

In 1978 Beeson and his colleagues issued "Aging and Medical Education," the first of a series of IoM studies that dealt with educating healthcare professionals in an aging society. Besides proposing aging-related materials for curricula, the report recommended upgrading the place of gerontology and geriatrics in U.S. academic medicine. Although geriatrics was an academic specialty in the United Kingdom, Beeson deemed elder care to be too broad to be handled by a few selected branches of medicine. Geriatrics was integral to most medical areas. To counter likely resistance, the report urged department chairs to secure the support of distinguished senior faculty willing to serve as role models, especially to train healthcare personnel to work with older patients in a multidisciplinary setting (Beeson, 1985; von Preyss-Friedman, 2009).

Not surprisingly, Butler found much to like in "Aging and Medical Education." He too opposed formalizing a geriatrics specialty. Medical schools should require basic and clinical courses as well as clinical clerkships and house staff training programs, he felt, in addition to offering materials on aging in continuing education curricula:

> Many of us were taught to find one or as few diagnoses as possible to explain a patient's symptoms. . . . Our professors frequently referred to this principle as William of Occam's razor. But as we grow older our bodies become more complex and more different. And it becomes much more difficult to identify and grapple successfully with the causes of an illness. Thus, we need more emphasis on the multiplicity and complexity of disease processes in the aged very early in our students' education and training.
>
> (BUTLER, 1979:904)

Faced with the aging of World War II personnel, the Veterans Administration (VA), noted Butler, did much to educate and train physicians in geriatric labs and clinics. Indeed, in 1978 the VA created a Geriatric Medicine Fellowship program to teach physicians to be mentors to medical students and residents. Two years later the VA introduced a Geriatric Psychiatry Fellowship program (Department of Veterans Affairs, 2008). Since these two programs offered the largest opportunities for geriatric training, NIA worked with the VA to do more.

To insinuate aging-related modules into medical-school curricula, Butler invited the deans of 126 U.S. allopathic medical schools to come to Bethesda to consider how to develop geriatric education. Roughly 30 deans promised to come. Although he persuaded few administrators, Butler told me that he judged the meeting a success because Dean Terry Rogers from the University of Hawaii sent a second-year medical student, Patricia Blanchette, who became a geriatrician and established a geriatrics department at her alma mater in 2002 (personal communication, January 3, 2010). Butler also promoted the idea of the "teaching nursing home," giving grants with discretionary funds to make teaching nursing homes the counterpart of teaching hospitals.

CONNECTING WITH POWER BROKERS

As an old-age advocate and political activist, Butler learned during the 1960s and early 1970s the importance of interacting with Washington's elite. With his boss's approval he took advantage of his position as head of NIA, his knowledge of aging, and his engaging manner as he worked on Capitol Hill. He assisted successive chairs of the Senate Special Committee on Aging. Butler already knew Sen. Frank Church (D-ID) from Vietnam activities; from 1971 to 1979 he advised Church and the staff of the Special Committee on Aging on housing and medical-care issues associated with amendments to the Social Security and Older Americans Acts. Similarly, between 1979 and 1981 he consulted Sen. Lawton Chiles (D-FL) on ways to provide health coverage for the uninsured. Butler had a warm relationship with Sen. John Heinz (R-PA), who held a powerful position on the Senate Finance Committee before becoming chair of the Special Committee on Aging from 1981 to 1987.

Butler also advised members of the House of Representatives, mainly in the House Select Committee on Aging, which was far larger than its Senate counterpart. Although it had no legislative power, the committee was influential during Butler's tenure at NIA because Claude Pepper (D-FL), who chaired the body in his seventies and eighties, was seasoned and savvy. Butler frequently met with Pepper's staff; he provided scientific evidence, for instance, that (with certain exceptions) existing age discrimination in employment laws were unnecessary and counterproductive.

Butler had many other friends on Capitol Hill. He remained close to Senator Eagleton. In 1977 he offered testimony on "the graying of nations" (1978) for Sen. John Glenn (D-OH). His ties with Sen. Daniel Patrick Moynihan (D-NY) deepened during the Social Security crisis of the early 1980s, as they did with Senator Heinz. On the House side Butler worked with Reps. Paul Rogers, an early supporter of NIA, and Joseph D. Early (D-MA). Some relations were strained. Butler did not like Rep. Daniel Flood (D-PA), who used his seniority on the House Appropriations Committee to constrain NIA's budget growth (Kashatus, 2010). And while Butler and Sen. Alan Cranston (D-CA) collaborated on health-care matters (such as supporting women's access to health care and supporting the rights of people with disabilities) and on establishing the Alliance for Aging Research (AAR), the men were wary (and rightly so) of each other's opinions concerning how far science could conquer disease, old age, and death (AAR, 2001).

Illustrative of Butler's influence on policy makers was his service to the National Commission on Social Security Reform, convened in 1981 to prevent the program from going bankrupt. This was the first time that the National Institute on Aging had been invited to contribute knowledge relevant to Social Security policy issues. The commission's executive director, Robert J. Myers, asked Butler, as NIA director, to focus on "the work ability of the aged population as it has changed over the years and as it might change in the future if mortality continues to decrease and life expectancy to increase" (Achenbaum, 1986; Butler, 1983a). Butler offered a detailed response. He noted the ethnic and racial diversity of the workforce in terms of health status, morbidity, and mortality rates as well as differences in gender-specific employment histories and functional capacities. "Retirement decisions are being made around the focal age points of 62, 65, and 68 without any real understanding of many impacts on human health and human performance," he concluded. "Biomedical *and* psychosocial factors need to be explored in studies of human performance" (1983a:428–29).

Nor did Butler restrict advice to elected leaders. Two surgeons general benefited from his services: NIA staff contributed to the work of Julius Richmond's *Healthy People*, which offered quantitative evidence to bolster public-health measures and recommend wise lifestyle choices for various age groups (Heinz Awards, 2008; U.S. HEW, 1979). Conversations with the NIA director influenced how Ronald Reagan's surgeon general, C. Everett Koop, MD, chose to advocate cost-effective ways to improve care of people who are disabled and older people (Koop, 1984). In addition Butler assisted Rosalyn Carter in preparing testimonies she delivered as First Lady as an honorary chair of the President's Commission on Mental Health and, after she left the White House, in establishing a program for mental-health advocacy through the Carter Center.

In some instances Butler acted as a mentor to associates in the network on aging. He assisted journalist Dan Perry, who often joined conversations about longevity and immortality that Senator Cranston had with Butler. Out of these talks emerged the idea for the Fund for Integrative Biomedical Research (FIBRE), which in 1986 led to the establishment of the Alliance for Aging Research, a nonprofit group that advocates that gerontological knowledge inform health policies. "I think the National Institute on Aging . . . deserves a huge amount of credit for trying to bring experts from around the country to really begin to build a sense of consensus . . . [that] lead to healthier aging across the population," Dan Perry, AAR's first director, declared. "I can't imagine anything that's more important to the United States, to Europe, to most of the developed world in the 21st century than to understand aging as a means to delay physiological and functional decline and to enhance the quality of life as long as possible for more people" (Perry, n.d.).

Butler connected with interesting people everywhere. Three examples suffice. First, he befriended Maggie Kuhn, who in 1970 convened what would become the Gray Panthers. Best known for her group's attention-grabbing tactics at the 1974 American Medical Association convention to protest the health-care industry, Kuhn regularly testified before the Senate Special Committee on Aging. In 1976 she paid a visit to NIA. Thereafter Butler worked with her to promote social security and fight ageism (Laursen, 2010). Second, while he doubted the effectiveness of an anti-aging formula known at Gerovital GH3, he nonetheless was in contact with its inventor, the Romanian biologist and physician Ana Aslan. Third, Butler, eager to give prominence to women's issues at NIA, invited Betty Friedan, author of the *Feminine Mystique* (1963), to Washington's Cosmos Club. Their collaboration blossomed when he moved to New York. He later encouraged her to write *Fountain of Age*; she also served as a director on the board of his International Longevity Center (Sinclair, 1989).

Furthermore, during his years at NIA Butler insisted on making media contacts and forging partnerships abroad. He put information about the National Institute on Aging in *Science*. He maintained warm ties with writers and editors at the *Washington Post*, and he reached out to Jack Rosenthal, a Pulitzer Prize–winning reporter, editor, and executive at the *New York Times* since 1969. He also cultivated relations with members of the Columbia School of Journalism and the John S. and James L. Knight Foundation. He assisted younger, politically astute journalists such as Paul Kleyman (Butler, personal communication, March 2010). On the international front he solicited information at the 1976 World Health Organization (WHO) to determine the number and scope of institutes abroad that had programs in the field of aging. This resulted in three meetings with research directors and a WHO publication that set the stage for collaborative projects to advance geriatrics, health promotion and disease prevention, epidemiological studies, and the sharing of resources (including animals and cells) and faculty and student exchanges (Butler, 1980; NIA, 1977).

Off duty Butler made gerontological insights accessible through mass media. In 1976, after conversations with the Planned Parenthood of America's Mary Steichen Calderone, he and his wife Myrna Lewis wrote *Sex After Sixty*. Despite the refusal of a Florida newspaper to advertise the book because it was "too prurient for the general public," it became a best seller. Over the next twenty-five years the book went through several editions, including (by 2002) a broader title, *The New Love and Sex After 60*. Butler and Lewis offered in dispassionate, often clinical, language advice to elders, be they single, gay, widowed or divorced. "People are always a little surprised that couples could write together and get along, but we did," Butler told a reporter. "She and I were intellectually close" (Hahn, 2005). Another best seller that Butler wrote with Lewis, *Aging and Mental Health*, appeared in revised editions in 1977 and 1982/1983, the latter with a foreword by *ABC News*'s Hugh Downs, who hosted the PBS series *Over Easy*. "This book, in its clear exposition of the difficulties and wide range of procedures through which meaningful improvement in the lot of our elders can be brought about," declared Downs, "shows age in the light in which any civilization ought to view it" (1983:ix).

% % % % %

Shortly before he left NIA in 1982 to become head of the Department of Geriatrics and Adult Development at the Mount Sinai School of Medicine in New York, Butler spoke to Janice Caldwell, former executive director of the Gerontological Society of America. "I am pleased that the Institute's very formulation in the Research on Aging Act spoke to the complexity of the human condition," Butler declared. "It did not make this a purely biomedical research institute but it made it biomedical, behavioral, and social" (Achenbaum & Albert, 1995:64–66; Butler, 1983b:8–12). Butler left for his successor, T. Franklin Williams, a 361-page update to *Our Future Selves*, including nearly 80 pages of references. *Toward an Independent Old Age: A National Plan for Research on Aging* (1982) demonstrated how far NIA had come in terms of breadth and society over Butler's six years as director. Williams, a distinguished clinician and geriatric administrator, shared Butler's vision and love of learning new things about age and aging (Williams, 1986:53).

Butler had ample reason to be pleased with his accomplishments, but he left behind much for Williams to do. And the political climate was shifting. Neoconservatives in the Reagan administration sought to curtail the rate of spending growth in Washington. This meant that there would be less discretionary money for new initiatives in aging that required federal oversight. Among his disappointments was that neither the public nor private sector "has really come to grips with the extraordinary change that's facing our population as a consequence of the increased numbers of older persons." So while he took pride in quadrupling his budget over six years (more, if one counts funds from collaborating with other institutes at Bethesda), NIA still accounted for only 2 percent of the NIH budget (Barfield, 1982:xiii, 1, 61; Butler, 1983b:8–9). Convinced that "almost every area will need more training support," Butler sought a bigger role for geriatrics in academic medicine (Butler, 1983b:11).

For the rest of his life, two hurdles frustrated Butler's efforts to realize his dream that NIA and other federal agencies would invest in old age in a manner commensurate with addressing the challenges and opportunities he associated with societal aging. On the one hand, gerontology remained peripheral to Big Science and vested interests in the policy arena. On the other hand, Butler's argument that basic research in aging was cost effective did not sway members of the emerging power elite who wanted to cut the size of Big Government, not add to its purview. There would be no constructive action, Butler acknowledged, until policy makers and the public got beyond ageism and neoconservatism sufficiently to embrace his vision of *Our Future Selves*. Ever the optimist and empiricist, however, he relished the intellectual challenge. As a private citizen he used his considerable powers of persuasion whenever and wherever possible.

six

EXPANDING THE SCOPE
OF GERIATRICS

Prior to 1978, wrote William R. Hazzard, geriatric education in postwar America "had no recognition as a specialty by the American Board of Internal Medicine and no designated training programs for faculty development or clinical geriatrics training" (John A. Harford Foundation, 2005). Hazzard created training programs at the University of Washington, Johns Hopkins, and Wake Forest schools of medicine, but he might have added that prior to 1978 there were no geriatrics departments in any U.S. medical school or model-care program. Nor was there a prescribed course of study for licensing nurses or credentialing social workers, dentists, and public health experts before the 1980s. Compared with Britain, where he had spent the 1977–78 year in a geriatrics department, Hazzard concluded that geriatric education lagged in the United States.

As director of the National Institute of Aging, Butler had expanded the scope of geriatrics. The Research on Aging Act of 1974 required NIA to "provide training and instruction and establish traineeships and fellowships, in the Institute and elsewhere" (National Research Council, 1976). Butler presented his aims in the first NIA blueprint, *Our Future Selves*

(1978): "The essential element . . . [is] a sufficient number of highly trained biologists, chemists, physicians, sociologists, psychologists, economists, and others—with long-range career commitment principally to research on the process of aging and the needs of the aged."

Butler proposed that, ideally, predoctoral and postdoctoral fellows be trained in interdisciplinary institutions that focused on age-related problems, such as studies on alcohol and aging conducted by gerontologists, biomathematicians, pharmacologists, physiologists, and psychologists; and multidisciplinary research on how medical, social, and economic support should be delivered to older Americans. "Such regional and university-based research centers would not only provide foci for the concentration of a small pool of first-class talent, but would also provide more effective training for students, as well as easier access to necessary resources at reduced costs" (34–35).

In his 1979 essay "Geriatrics and Internal Medicine," one of his most cited articles, Butler argued that the emphasis on pathologic aging rather than normal senescence precludes "appropriate training . . . to ensure the kinds of clinical practice and research that form the basis of good health and health delivery system." Clinical medicine's preoccupation with the irreversible aspects of disease processes in late life, he believed, had thwarted the appeal of geriatrics to health-care professionals.

> If medical education is to respond adequately to the growing number of citizens encompassed by the field of geriatric medicine, it must intensify its commitment to the special health and health-related problems of the elderly at every level, from student to certified specialist. . . . As our country recognizes this new-found reservoir of strength and capability, we in the medical profession should continue our self-evaluation to determine how we can most effectively contribute to improving the lives of the elderly, perhaps our greatest national resource.
>
> (BUTLER, 1979:903, 907–8; SEE ALSO SCHAFER, 2009:2–4)

Producing more doctors versed in geriatric principles would require a major infusion of federal training funds. The expenditure was easy to justify, argued Butler. The investment would enable older Americans in better care to contribute more as a result of improved health-care delivery. Having observed and studied clinical experiences, he thought that this proposal was a cost-effective way to address population aging.

There were at least three obstacles. First, there were not many physician scientists trained like Butler. Second, applying "Occam's razor" in clinical training—teaching medical students how to determine the least number of factors necessary to diagnose a patient's malady and to develop a treatment plan—was antithetical to best practices in geriatrics. Symptoms grow more complex as bodies age, Butler noted, and "it becomes much more difficult to identify and grapple successfully with the causes of an illness" (904–5). A third factor was ageism. Unlike future pediatricians who see healthy babies and talk to their parents, few medical students had chances to interact with healthily aging men and women. Medical students rarely had the time or inclination to listen to older people's health self-assessments or desires for better vision or hearing, muscle strength, or productivity. There were fewer miracle drugs for elders compared with remedies for the diseases of childhood and middle age. "The negative associations . . . may serve to reinforce latent or overt prejudices and establish a pattern of lifelong rejection of the elderly" (905–6).

To surmount difficulties, Butler recommended that training people to care for the aged be integrated into all phases of medical education, particularly in primary-care specialties. He did not advocate that a distinctive specialty be designated geriatrics. Nor, he emphasized, were general practitioners and specialists older people's only caregivers. "We should stress the 'team approach' . . . of dentists, podiatrists, nurses, social workers, physical and occupational therapists, nutritionists, psychologists, physician's assistants, and others working together under the leadership of the physician—to provide the best possible care for the older patient" (905–6). Butler also intended to augment continuing-education and research opportunities to physicians in practice who wished to focus on elder care.

Hazzard shared Butler's vision. "Geriatrics may be the last haven of the general physician, not only because such complex and subtle judgements are required but because the more technically oriented subspecialist is less attracted to the patient with multiple problems which blur diagnostic borders and may even inhibit aggressive diagnosis and treatment" (Hazzard, 1979:141–42). Like Butler, Hazzard realized that inducements—first-rate facilities, financial resources, and consultations with other health professionals—were essential to promoting geriatrics, lest an inferior sub-specialty result.

Many structural aspects of U.S. medical care seemed conducive to promoting geriatrics as Butler and Hazzard proposed. America had plenty of excellent hospitals in which to initiate programs. And there was a critical mass of health-care professionals—assuming the capacity and flexibility to (re)deploy members of the workforce—to care for older people, historically an underserved segment of the population. Finally, all the relevant indicators (public-health interventions, research advances, and technological innovations) signaled improvements in Americans' health conditions overall—whether outcomes were measured by falling age-adjusted death rates, declines in deaths from major diseases and disability, or improved infant and maternal mortality statistics (Greenberg & Fein, 1999:10–17; Rogers, 1978:54–55).

Both pioneers underestimated the difficulties, however. There were only 20 required geriatric rotations among the 753 accredited residency programs in internal medicine and family medicine in 1977–78; just 45 of the 8,795 continuing education courses listed in the directory of the *Journal of the American Medical Association* dealt with geriatrics (Butler, 1979:905–6). Conditions abroad were not terribly encouraging. Having called the United Kingdom "the Mecca of geriatrics," Hazzard went on to rue "the descending spiral which has plagued geriatrics" there (1979:141–42; see also Taggart, 1981:69–72). Intramural politics in academic medicine, institutional constraints, and fiscal exigencies nationally and locally conspired to thwart efforts to expand geriatrics.

THE STATE OF AMERICAN MEDICINE CIRCA 1980

American medicine was undergoing a transformation at the very moment that Butler and others advanced their geriatric mandate. Costs were escalating. Public and private insurance did not cover all fees to visit physicians. Hospital-care costs soared at twice the rate of other commodities. Health-care disparities in services were widening by race and region. Criticisms about poor management mirrored complaints about administrative indifference over the care being delivered (Rogers, 1978:10, 12).

Furthermore, the proportion of general practitioners fell from 64 percent to 24 percent between 1949 and 1973. The decline affected physician–patient relationships in three ways. First, general practitioners faced "the hazard of having [their] expertise atrophy from disuse" since they rarely treated patients with complex issues. Second, some, like Ivan Illich in *Medical Nemesis* (1975), flatly questioned doctors' efficacy. "Many people felt that physicians and other health personnel lacked interest and/or skill in understanding and coping with the anxiety, despair, and loneliness that often accompany illness" (McDermott, 1980:124; Rogers, 1977:85, 87; 1978:10, 84;). Third, general practitioners long had been the frontline doctors most likely to see older patients.

By the 1980s divisions sharpened within the profession among those in academic settings, office-based practitioners working alone or in a group practice, doctors in rural areas, and foreign-trained physicians. The presence of more women in medical schools and specialties challenged androcentric norms in the profession, but minorities remained underrepresented except in low-paying jobs. While the American Medical Association, founded in 1847, was the profession's chief bargaining agent, less than half of all physicians were members. No wonder Paul Starr claimed in *The Social Transformation of American Medicine* that "the 1960s and 1970s broke down the uniformity and cohesiveness of the profession" (1982:90, 427). Patients expected physicians to be up-to-date with technology, pharmacology, and other interventions. General practitioners acceded and referred patients to specialists—as long as they were not cut out of the system (Abbott, 1988; Anlyan & Graves, 1973:x, 9; DeGroot, 1966:243).

The dominance of specialists in the medical profession fragmented health-care delivery. Since its founding in 1933, the physician-led American Board of Medical Specialties (ABMS) had sought to assist Member Boards to develop professional and educational standards with which to evaluate candidates for certification in any given specialty. By 1980 there were twenty-two Member Boards overseeing examinations in roughly 140 specialties and subspecialties (ABMS, n.d.; Cooper, 2008). Stakeholders, from solo practitioners to board-certified pathologists, wished to protect prerogatives, including hospital privileges and access to beds. This sparked resistance to any proposed changes in the status quo that threatened people's income and identity. The proliferation of specialists among allied health professionals resulted in competition for shared resources as well as duplication of skills and tests. The geographic misallocation of physicians added to competitive pressures (Califano, 1979:19).

In this changing milieu, experts perceived the present and future needs of older patients through very different lenses. The problems of the elderly poor (along with those of poor children, rural dwellers, chronically ill people, and people with disabilities) topped the agenda of the Robert Wood Johnson Foundation (RWJF): population aging "will alter the character of families and communities," declared David Rogers, who had been dean of the Johns Hopkins Medical School before serving as head of RWJF from 1971 to 1986. "It will add to the number of individuals with chronic disease, and it will add to the problems of how we plan for the support of those no longer able to care for themselves" (Rogers, 1977:90; 1978:32–40).

Others felt that existing arrangements could accommodate current demands by elderly patients. This camp questioned whether the aged poor would or could utilize resources if they had greater access. They noted, for instance, the widespread ignorance among older people about mental-health facilities in New York (DeGroot, 1967; Elinson, Padila, & Perkins, 1967:10, 132).

Still others, like Butler, decried gaps in coverage. He also documented and excoriated ageism in virtually all health-care facilities that (under) served the elderly (Butler, 1975b:4–5). Surgeon General C. Everett Koop opined that crafting "a philosophy of aging for the public health professions" might help to reconcile "different perspectives, with differing, value-laden data, and with differing concepts" (1983:203).

According to experts, the future of U.S. medicine, including the fate of geriatrics, would rest in academic medical centers. There were 114 such centers in 1977, which competed for scientists and recruited students for their research institutes, biological laboratories, and ambulatory clinics in affiliated hospitals. "With the development of scientific medicine, the hospital, especially the teaching and research hospital, has come to be the frontier of medical knowledge and of the technology of its successful application (Cole & Lipton, 1977; Parsons & Platt, 1973:238; Rogers, 1978; Smythe, 1967; Wilson, 1968). As medical centers expanded in size and complexity, they grew autonomous from one another as well as from their home base: deans, department chairs, and well-funded investigators could do what they wished as long as centers remained accredited. Medicare, enacted in 1965, became the major financial catalyst for the growth of U.S. academic medical centers. Many tapped this resource to advance family medicine. Administrators in teaching hospitals had considerable discretionary freedom over such funds because the federal government was forbidden to supervise operations or personnel selection (Ginzberg, 2000:29, 50; Ginzberg, Berliner, & Ostow, 1993:32; Ginzberg & Dutka, 1989:5; Graham & Diamond, 1997:209–10; Rogers, 1978:80–81; Thomas, 1987).

Then, in the late 1970s, changing economic conditions caught most professionals by surprise. Double-digit inflation dashed hopes for continued prosperity. Policy makers worried about the federal deficit. Administrators could not control hospital budgets. There were deep layoffs and cutbacks in New York's health sector as city officials staved off bankruptcy. No new acute beds were added, despite a succession of health crises—the AIDS epidemic in the early 1980s, followed by a crack pandemic, and growing numbers of homeless persons, many discharged from mental institutions. At the federal level politicians were recommending larger deductibles and higher copayments for older people to avoid a depletion of the Medicare trust fund (Ginzberg, 1985:169–70; Ginzberg, Berliner, & Ostow, 1993:1, 15–16, 20, 38, 198).

SPEARHEADING GERIATRICS AT
MOUNT SINAI MEDICAL CENTER

Mount Sinai Hospital had been a venerable New York City institution for more than a century before its trustees established an academic medical center in 1963. Members of the English, Portuguese, and German Jewish elite in 1855 opened the forty-five-bed Jews' Hospital (as it was originally known), supporting it handsomely through benefit dinners, private donations, and bequests. To secure eligibility for public funding, the facility was renamed in 1866 and abandoned its sectarian charter—though its population base remained primarily Jewish. Six years later, relocating from West 28th Street to Lexington Avenue, Mount Sinai nearly tripled its capacity. After the turn of the century, it began to hire caseworkers to provide social services. Trustees tried to balance its mission of treating patients (mainly Russian Jews) with delivering health care that met the research and clinical objectives of medical specialists (Mount Sinai Medical Center, n.d.; Rosenberg, 1987:314–15, 418nn7, 13).

In the 1950s the hospital decided to build a university of health sciences. The trustees envisioned a first-rate medical school supported by Mount Sinai's teaching hospital, graduate schools of biological and physical sciences, and a center for health-care research. The medical school was authorized in 1963, a dean was appointed two years later, and students were admitted in 1968 ("Mount Sinai School of Medicine," n.d; Smythe, 1967:994). Mount Sinai had strong support from organized medicine, NIH research funding, and philanthropists.

In less than a decade the medical school was ranked in twenty-first place, just above NYU's medical school. Yet it was not all smooth sailing. In 1973 a strike by hospital union Local 1199, which was supported by medical students, had long-lasting repercussions (Cole & Lipton, 1977:669; Ludmerer, 1999:239). Mount Sinai's plant was outmoded: like the New York and Presbyterian hospitals, it used facilities constructed in the 1930s. Parking difficulties, busy traffic, and fear of street crime diminished Mount Sinai's appeal (Ginzberg, 1985:120).

In response, the hospital unveiled a threefold strategy: First, it closed some outpatient clinics, limited services to those in narrowly defined catchment areas, and referred patients it did not want to public hospitals. Second, it advertised its physician referral services through a multimedia campaign to attract more patients (Ginzberg, Berliner, & Ostow, 1993:23; Johnson, 1982). Third, it cultivated markets, including geriatrics, where prospects for growth looked bright.

Mount Sinai already was a pioneer in aging. The father of U.S. geriatrics, Dr. I. L. Nascher, had been chief of its Outpatient Department. Nascher published *Geriatrics: The Diseases of Old Age and Their Treatment, Including Physiological Old Age, Home and Institutional Care, and Medico-Legal Relations* in 1914. Abraham Jacobi, who in his introduction to the book linked geriatrics to pediatrics (his specialty), helped Nascher to formulate subsequent life-course perspectives on gerontology.

In 1921 Mount Sinai physician Frederic Zeman developed a model for elder care through the Home for Aged and Infirm Hebrews (later named the Jewish Home and Hospital), where he served as medical director for forty-five years. Dr. Zeman's efforts enabled Leslie Libow, MD, to create the first geriatric fellowship, which trained residents working in acute outpatient departments and long-term care facilities. This initiative subsequently expanded into a residency program at Elmhurst, a teaching facility of Mount Sinai, which was certified by the American Board of Internal Medicine. In 1979 Mount Sinai recruited Fred Sherman, MD, to establish a geriatrics division within the Department of Internal Medicine. A year later an Interdisciplinary Geriatric Consult Team began, consisting of a physician, nurse, and social worker (Mount Sinai Medical Center, n.d.).

Mount Sinai's trustees invited NIA director Butler to tell them how to launch a first-rate geriatrics center. The board (which included Dr. Lewis Thomas and Robert Rubin, a senior partner at Goldman Sachs and future U.S. treasury secretary under President Bill Clinton) was so impressed by Butler and his ideas that it cabled him the day after his visit, inviting him to move to New York to spearhead the nation's first Department of Geriatrics. Butler hesitated. Despite cuts in NIH's growth rates during the Reagan administration, Butler enjoyed his job and figured he could probably hold it indefinitely. He and his wife liked Washington, especially their home on Huntington Avenue. Indeed, he loved his residence so much that he invited Dr. Thomas Chalmers, Mount Sinai's president, to see where and how he lived. Although he could not replicate Butler's gardens, Chalmers did promise Bob and Myrna a spacious apartment overlooking Central Park West.

Realizing that a move from the public to the private sector in economically turbulent times was risky, Butler composed a twelve-page memorandum that mapped out what he needed to develop a center of excellence. Acknowledging the impact of "attacks on current reimbursement patterns," he sought ways to relieve the problem of "blocked beds" at the hospital. "My proposals will help prepare Mount Sinai to meet demands for economy in the most effective and humane ways" (Butler, n.d.:2, 7).

If he were to be given $3 million over each of the next three years, Butler predicted, he would have a program in place within five years with a flow of 2,000 new and 4,000 follow-up patients through a diagnosis-and-referral unit; there would be 6,500 patients a year admitted to clinical geriatrics. He promised to design a curriculum based on geriatric principles and practices for *all* medical students. He envisioned an "aggressive" research program in three laboratories: (1) Cell Biology and Aging, (2) Homeostasis/Regulatory Aspects of Aging, and particularly (3) Neurosciences and Dementias of Aging. The research program, he reckoned, would require 5,000 square feet of laboratory space, nine senior investigators (Butler identified Caleb Finch, Jeffrey Halter, and John Rowe as likely candidates), six fellows, and twelve technicians (n.d., appendix A). Start-up would run $2.5 million, with $750,000 in annual operating and supply costs.

Butler's research agenda—coupled with demonstration models of geriatric inpatient and outpatient care—aimed to insinuate geriatrics and gerontology into all aspects of professional education, scientific investigations, and policy and planning activities on the Mount Sinai campus and at its affiliated institutions. Among other initiatives, Butler wanted to create hospice services with the Department of Neoplastic Diseases. "The major organizational instrument of this plan is a Mount Sinai Department of Geriatrics and Human Development. It will include an Institute on Health and Socioeconomic Policy for Aging [which would focus on productive aging], a major long-term care and rehabilitative project at the Jewish Home and Home and Hospital for Aged, and strong education" (11, 13).

Butler wanted Mount Sinai's new hospital, which was under construction while he was being recruited, to "be designed with elderly patients in mind, and services within it should be so oriented." A Geriatric Assessment and Referral Service would handle diagnoses, treatment plans, and follow-up consultations for patients drawn from the community, region, and nation. The Geriatric Clinical Demonstration Unit would attend to referrals from other departments, enabling students and residents to deal "with the classic type of geriatric patients—individuals having multiple problems, including those in frail health, suffering from drug toxicity, nutritional ailments, and psychosocial difficulties." To this end, in addition to a unit with twenty beds and appropriate specialist and nursing support, Butler requested a cluster of four surgical beds, as well as an additional three or four beds reserved for the Department of Geriatrics in the Mount Sinai General Clinical Research Center. In some cases Butler's staff would coordinate health-care delivery with the Jewish Home and Hospital for Aged, the Bronx VA, and the Hospitals for Joint Diseases. For an analog to a Well-Baby Center, Butler proposed a Wellness Clinic where community-based elders would get low-cost screening and help for families dealing with Alzheimer's (6, 7–9, 12).

Butler emphasized multidisciplinary, trans-professional educational initiatives. To train medical students, and to satisfy "the goal of disseminating geriatric knowledge among the specialties and among the primary care fields, notably internal medicine," Butler requested that he be allocated twenty hours during the first two years of the medical curriculum, a four-week rotation in the third year, and an elective in geriatrics available to all fourth-year students. In addition, he proposed an MD-PhD program to prepare physician scientists for careers in academic gerontology, a geriatric medical residency program, and a two-year medical geriatric fellowship program for candidates board-eligible in internal medicine and in other fields. He indicated that he would welcome trainees from public health, neurology, family practice, rehabilitation medicine, psychiatry, and other health fields to train under his unit's supervision.

Besides training undergraduate and graduate medical students, Butler intended to develop continuing-education materials for physicians and intensive courses for associate professors in medical schools that wished to add geriatrics to their curricula. He wanted Mount Sinai to be a hub for training professionals who worked with older people (12). Through the Brookdale Center for Continuous Education, courses would be offered for nurses, nursing aides, social workers, families, and individuals.

Proud of the media attention he had generated for NIA, Butler proposed three information outlets. First, he wanted a scientific information office, as he had in Bethesda, to prepare materials on aging for professional and lay audiences. Second, he intended to write a nationally syndicated column on aging. Third, the department would have a library on gerontology and geriatrics to serve as a resource for the city.

One request was nonnegotiable: "The Department will require a strong foundation in specific agreements as to funds, staff, facilities, and policy directions," Butler asserted. "The Department will express leadership in large measure as a collaborator, convener, and catalyst of activities within the medical school and teaching hospital" (4; see also Butler & Gleason, 1985:568). Instead of operating autonomously, as did heads of medical units elsewhere, the Department of Geriatrics and Human Development that Butler proposed would be recognized as "the essential colleague" to all departments and programs collaboratively assessing needs and achieving outcomes "in the interests of the most humane, effective, and cost-efficient treatment of elderly patients." Dr. Chalmers agreed to the arrangement. Butler also stipulated that funds be available to cover joint ventures and dual appointments.

Expecting geriatrics to grow from a position of strength, Robert Butler did his best to guarantee a prominent leadership role at Mount Sinai. He wanted to serve on the medical school's curriculum committee. In addition to having *"sole control"* over designated endowments, the department would be "the acknowledged focal point" in obtaining public and private funds for research on aging, teaching, and service. It would control its promotions and determine how attending physicians spent their time. In return, Mount Sinai would reap enormous benefits:

> I will bring to bear my knowledge, experience, and contacts in the interests of a bold, comprehensive Mount Sinai program in geriatrics in accord with the intentions of the admirable Mount Sinai prospectus on developing national leadership in geriatrics. My plan has the best potential of attracting topflight scientists, clinicians, and other experts to Mount Sinai for what surely will be regarded as a bellwether effort to gear American medicine to the needs of an aging population.
>
> (1)

Butler knew that he was asking a lot, but he also knew he had a lot to offer to Mount Sinai. The trustees considered his requests reasonable enough to confirm promises in writing before he signed on. He figured that he would have to compete with other chairs for increments to his budget or, in dire straits, to fend off cutbacks. Looking back, he admitted to me that he did not fully anticipate the turf battles he would face.

Butler displayed great vision in launching geriatrics at Mount Sinai. His leadership inspired confidence among colleagues and community leaders. The Gerald and May Ellen Ritter Foundation underwrote the department; the Brookdale Foundation funded his chair. In roughly a year, Geriatrics had six faculty members and eight postgraduate fellows. Mount Sinai did not honor one request: Butler wanted his unit to be called the Department of Geriatrics and Human Development, to underscore a life-course approach. Instead, the objection of the chair of the Department of Pediatrics prevailed, and the unit was designated "Geriatrics and Adult Development." Still, Butler's requests paid off. Chalmers made room in the medical curriculum for mandatory geriatric instruction and, with the trustees' support, authorized a research program in the biomedical sciences. Four accomplishments merit particular note.

First, as he had done at NIA, Robert Butler attracted and nurtured first-rate talent. Drs. Christine K. Cassel and Diane Meier called him in 1982 from the Oregon Health Sciences Center to see if they could join him at Mount Sinai. Although she stayed only three years, Cassel returned to chair the Department of Geriatrics from 1995 to 2002 (Cassel, 2005). Meier remained at Mount Sinai, where she created a renowned program in palliative care, received major funding from NIA, and was awarded a Mac-Arthur "Genius" fellowship. Besides making a considerable number of media appearances, she coauthored with Cassel the fourth edition of *Geriatric Medicine: An Evidence-Based Approach* (Cassel et al., 2003).

Other colleagues' contributions enhanced Mount Sinai's strength in geriatrics. Barbara Paris, MD, a geriatrics fellow (1983–1986) now routinely listed as a top doctor in the United States, became Butler's personal physician. Howard M. Fillit, MD, a geriatrician and neuroscientist, treated Estée Lauder while a fellow at Mount Sinai; he later became founding director of the Institute for the Study of Aging, a Lauder foundation. In addition, two NIA stalwarts—Mal Schecter and Judy Howe—relocated to Mount Sinai to head communications and departmental administration, respectively.

Second, Butler established at Mount Sinai the start-of-the-art geriatric-care continuum that he had in mind at NIA. "Affiliated with a university, teaching nursing homes would generate new knowledge about diseases affecting the elderly," Butler opined. "Their effectiveness, quality, ability to attract and hold professions, and public image would thereby be improved" (Butler, 1981:1437). With Leslie Libow, chief of medical services at the Jewish Home and Hospital and a professor of geriatrics at Mount Sinai, who had helped to prepare the memorandum of understanding, Butler nurtured a site through which roughly two hundred geriatric fellows rotated.

In addition, Butler established with the help of Mrs. Avery Fisher a Healthy Elderly program for men and women over sixty near Mount Sinai at the 92d Street Y. This wellness center featured intergenerational programs in the arts and culture, as well as facilities for improving health and promoting fitness. The partnership between the Y and Mount Sinai benefited both organizations by fostering positive images of aging.

Third, Butler garnered the interest and support of philanthropists and foundations. Betty Wold Johnson, through the Robert Wood Johnson Foundation, contributed an endowed professorship in neurobiology and underwrote a laboratory for aging. William Golden, a Mount Sinai trustee who had been active in recruiting Butler, helped to find money to establish the first inpatient unit at the medical center. Engaging New York celebrities paid off, eventually leading (among other things) to the creation of the Martha Stewart Center for Living at Mount Sinai, which offered community referrals, caregiver support, medical care, and programs for healthy living. In addition, Butler and his colleagues secured NIH grants and research projects through agencies in New York City and New York State (Rosenzweig & Turlington, 1982:20). Butler managed to mix private and public funding sources in a way that afforded him discretionary freedom.

Finally, thanks to Butler's reputation and perspicacity, the Department of Geriatrics and Adult Development quickly became the model for other medical centers to emulate. "The creation of an independent department at Mount Sinai Medical Center may represent a milestone in American medical association," opined Dr. Paul Beeson, author of "The Institute of Medicine Report on Aging and Medical Education" (1985:482). Officers of the John A. Hartford Foundation (2005) credited the department with being a model for six other departments of geriatrics across the nation and curricular initiatives at 105 other medical schools. "We will be proud of these accomplishments and leave them to our children," Butler wrote in 1984. "They will say we knew how to age well" (1984:16).

Despite this promising start, things unfortunately began to unravel. Butler (1985:568) admitted early in his tenure that it was "certainly the hardest job I have ever had." Chalmers left his position as president and dean of Mount Sinai School of Medicine in 1983 to become chairman of the board of the Dartmouth-Hitchcock Medical Center in New Hampshire (Fein, 1995). Without his friend and colleague at the helm, Butler had to deal with a new president (James Glenn, a urologist who had been dean of Emory University School of Medicine), whose chief responsibility was to raise at least $110 million to renovate and rejuvenate Mount Sinai's physical plant. The new dean, reproductive endocrinologist Nathan Kase, was unsympathetic to the geriatric initiative (Hartocollis, 2010). Nor did the appointment in 1988 of a Butler protégé, John W. Rowe, to be chief executive officer improve the situation much. Preoccupied with fiscal issues and community relations and wishing to capitalize on licenses and patents, Dr. Rowe sought to make ties with businesses, as did other academic entrepreneurs at the time (Altbach, Berdahl, & Gumport, 2005:124; Wilson, 1983:102; see also "John W. Rowe," 2010). In the late 1990s he successfully affiliated Mount Sinai with New York University, which created the largest academic medical center in the city.

Butler no longer had a superior like Chalmers who advocated for aging. Glenn and Kase worried that Mount Sinai might become too associated with geriatrics and old age, which seems an odd concern since at the time the city's population over sixty-five exceeded one million (Weinberg, 1995:290–96). Furthermore, Butler had to compete with other departments, which resented that the newcomer had claims to limited resources in hard times. Strong chairs "'stuck to knitting,' with all the limitations and benefits that such a strategy brings" (Ginzberg, Berliner, & Ostow, 1993:26; see also Cole, Barber, & Graubard, 1994:105; Heyssel et al., 1984:1477–80).

Butler considered leaving Mount Sinai on several occasions. He was invited to succeed his friend James Birren as head of the Andrus Gerontology Center at the University of Southern California. He was a strong contender to head the American Association of Retired Persons. Senator David Pryor (D-AR) supported him to become director of the National Institutes of Health in the Clinton administration. He was also recommended to become the nation's first assistant secretary for aging, a position that went to his friend, Fernando Torres-Gil.

Other options presented themselves. Butler was dissuaded from politics by Democratic Party leaders in New York. At Mount Sinai he had served on corporate boards such as Neurogen Corporation and Bio Time, Inc., as well as nonprofits such as the American Federation for Aging Research and the Kronos Longevity Research Institute. George Soros invited him to become more involved with Soros's Death in America project. Butler was well positioned to join well-paying boards and expand his consulting beyond advising the Donald W. Reynolds Foundation. In any event, he was quite content enjoying New York's cultural life and traveling abroad with Myrna Lewis.

INTRODUCING NEW IDEAS ABOUT
"PRODUCTIVE AGING"

Professionally the extent to which Butler wished to redirect geriatrics is evident in "A Generation at Risk," an essay written for the Hogg Foundation for Mental Health, where he situates concerns for *Our Future Selves* squarely on the baby boom cohort. Butler discounted forecasts of generational conflict between older whites and younger minorities, yet "to minimize dependency and maximize productivity, our society will have to spur institutional change" (1984:4–5; see also Longman, 1987; Peterson & Howe, 1988; Pifer & Bronte, 1986). It is worth noting that here and elsewhere he did not dwell on physical limitations and other liabilities increasingly likely to occur in people over age seventy-five. Instead he wrote about a Geriatric Gap that hindered "our knowledge of aging and disease processes in relation to practical decisions important in population aging" (1984:11).

In his opinion, those "practical decisions," it would become clear over time, were premised less on the familiar litany of the deficits of age and more on failures to harness the assets of late life, resources scarcely appreciated by his contemporaries. So, in agreeing to plan and chair the 1983 Salzburg Seminar, an intensive colloquium inviting fifty people to focus on a contemporary problem, Butler elaborated a theme he had articulated at NIA and Mount Sinai: he "urged that we move away from the popular concepts of dependence, long-term care, and costs of old age (all admittedly important) to a largely undeveloped topic, that of productivity in old age. . . . A major task is to reevaluate the very meaning of productivity. We cannot be satisfied with prevailing conceptions." Health and productivity wax and wane together over the life course, he asserted. "The unproductive human is at a higher risk of illness and economic dependency and the sick person is limited in productivity and is, therefore, at higher risk of dependency" (Butler & Gleason, 1985:xi, 8, 11, 14). This assessment was valid, of course: disease and misfortune can strike individuals at any age.

Butler was struggling to create a new vision of aging. That he gave short shrift to the cumulative loss of autonomy and capacities that can occur with advancing years is not surprising. Throughout the twentieth century geriatricians and gerontologists had endeavored to disentangle "normal" aging from various pathologies. What merits attention is that Butler was not alone in his effort to turn conventional wisdom on its head by offering scientific perspectives on productive aging.

Salzburg participants amplified Butler's call to vitalize older people's potentialities and capacities. Dr. Alvar Svanborg, a geriatrician at the University of Gothenberg, Sweden, deplored the way his colleagues misdiagnosed and overtreated patients over seventy: "Activity is much more feasible for elderly people than we assume, that activity is salubrious, and we should identify and eliminate societal barriers to it" (Butler & Gleason, 1985:21, 88, 91). James Birren, distinguishing among biological, social and anthropological, and psychological theories of aging, reminded participants that "humans have evolved with a large capacity for unique adaptations to environmental demands," sufficient for constructive activities (32). To achieve productive aging across generations, Betty Friedan urged colleagues to "integrate female strengths and male strengths into the human strengths of flexibility, intuition, and wisdom—the fruits of age" (103).

Mal Schecter, Butler's NIA and Mount Sinai colleague, detected a paradigm shift in the making: "The Fellows at Salzburg found that they had to test their own perceptions of aging, health, and productivity before undertaking the emerging task of constructing principles for new activities and attitudes" (123). For productive engagement to promote healthful aging, there had to be policies in place that encouraged older people to remain active. It was not enough to underwrite remedial interventions to secure "mere survival" for senior citizens, argued Butler. Every segment of society—especially health professionals and idea brokers—had to rethink stereotypes of age and capitalize on the strengths of the new old.

Over time, frustrated by the resistance of middle-aged and younger Americans to his ideas about health and productivity, Butler occasionally revealed pessimism. Asked in 1996 whether Americans were "anywhere near the progress you called for 20 years ago," Butler expressed concern about the prospects of baby boomers in old age:

I think the baby boomers and Generation X are very much at-risk, because a
lot of the privately-sponsored social experimentation will be practiced on
them, without much recourse to government. . . . They will prove to be the
transformational generation, and it may be 2030 before these issues begin to
work themselves out. Until then, I'm afraid we're in for a dark period. Of
course I could be wrong. And I wouldn't mind being wrong.

(FEIN, 1994; PECK, 1996)

Filling geriatric gaps and promoting productive aging were not novel strategies. More than ever, however, they had become cost-effective and prudent, Butler declared repeatedly—and, he admitted, often futilely.

Before the National Bipartisan Commission on the Future of Medicare,
for example, Butler argued that "delaying dysfunction is important when
we consider productivity. . . . It does not seem reasonable and economically
sustainable to have 65 million skilled and educated Baby Boomers sitting
idle. When older persons remain active in the work force they contribute to
a productive economy" (Butler, 1998b). Investing in geriatric training and
research on productive aging "would take only a modest investment to reap
benefits in cost containment and in an improved quality of life." He proposed that Medicare's General Education fund be used to train the three
thousand physicians that he estimated were needed to serve as geriatric
leaders. While he had the floor, he went on to urge NIA researchers to integrate biological and clinical investigations to pursue more assiduously issues in dementia and frailty.

As is true of most advisory councils, the bipartisan body limited its attention to the fiscal crisis at hand. The commission issued recommendations concerning Medicare coverage, solvency, and financing. It elected not
to widen its purview and take up the broad issues that Butler had laid out
for consideration.

Scholars grasped the significance of "productive aging," however. The
Center for Social Development at Washington University's George Warren
Brown School of Social Work sponsored a symposium in the late 1990s to
which it invited biomedical researchers, social scientists, and experts in the

humanities. "Productive aging would appear to be in the best interests of both society and the individual," Butler wrote in *Productive Aging* (Morrow-Howell, Hinterlong, & Sherraden, 2001:v). "Investments must be made today" (see also Butler & Osako, 1990; Kerschner & Pegues, 1998; Wheeler, 2009; Zelewski & Butrica, 2007).

To undercut parochialism in U.S. policy circles, Butler insisted that researchers, educators, and practitioners track global developments in aging. "We must borrow the best from overseas," he recommended. "Virtually every nation is faced with the same challenge: to prepare individuals and societies for the extraordinary human achievement—the revolution of longevity in the 20th century, which will become all the more marked in the 21st" (Butler & Osako, 1990).

Not only did Butler incorporate global perspectives into his ideas about productive aging, as we shall see in chapter 7, but he also became more forthright about the vulnerabilities of late life. He explicitly took into account frailty in relation to productivity with his former student, Howard Fillit, MD. "Societal strategies should include investigations of a 'biocultural' approach with population-based interventions that enable the 'fourth age' to be amenable to successful aging," Fillit and Butler recommended. Well aware of frailty's comorbidity with physical disorders and functional impairment, they urged researchers to focus on the psychological manifestations of vulnerability that resulted from a "frailty identity crisis." They proposed cognitive behavioral theory to remedy older people's atrophied sense of the future. "Volunteering and the creation of societal approaches to promote quality of life and independence in frail individuals should also be explored" (Fillit & Butler, 2009:351).

Thus Butler acknowledged the magnitude and distinctiveness of conditions manifest in "the Fourth Age," a term other investigators used to describe a segment of the life course when older persons no longer can maintain earlier levels of independence associated with healthy aging. Yet Butler did not want health-care professionals to be complacent in attending to those with diminishing capacity. Science and technology had done much to eliminate or ameliorate maladies once considered inevitable and untreatable. More advances were forthcoming. In his opinion geriatricians should "promote social alternatives to passive acceptance of frailty" (Fillit & Butler, 2009:351). In addition, grounding his hope that gerontologists and geriatricians would grasp the "big picture," Butler presupposed that peers would be knowledgeable about fast-breaking biomedical developments in aging.

Recent developments in basic research, he felt, were paramount in training professionals for clinical practice with elders. So in 1987, with three former NIA colleagues (Huber Warner, Richard L. Sprott, and Edward L. Schneider), he edited *Modern Biological Theories of Aging*. "It is time to evaluate contemporary theories of aging, clarify our state of knowledge, and encourage new research and new researchers," Butler declared in his foreword. "There are also important social, cultural, and economic reasons for expanding research to understand the underlying mechanisms of aging" (Butler, 1987:vii). *Modern Biological Theories of Aging* analyzed theories that remained robust. Meanwhile scientists continued to disentangle time-dependent factors and environmental conditions as they probed people's susceptibility to disease as they aged.

Butler (with twenty-two coauthors) updated this assessment of biogerontology fifteen years later in a special report on "The Aging Factor in Health and Disease: The Promise of Basic Research on Aging" (Butler et al., 2003). Here he stressed interventions to prevent or retard deleterious aspects of aging while improving people's quality of life amid striking increases in human life expectancy. "The conviction that basic research on aging is underfunded comes from the recognition that there are many unanswered questions about the basic mechanisms of aging, and that the answers to these questions may give us powerful insights about aging and the treatment of age-related diseases." Of the total amount of money the United States expended for health services for the aged, less than 1 percent was spent on research on aging.

Butler's case for geriatrics not only rested on his philosophy of science but also jibed with his administrative expertise. He connected investing in basic research, training health-care professionals, and promoting productive aging: "Any delay or reduction in age-related disability and disease will increase the number of years of healthy life and is a worthy goal. To facilitate such progress in understanding aging, there is a critical need not only for increased funding for aging research, but also funding for research infrastructure in the form of equipment and trained personnel" (Butler et al., 2003:110). Well-trained health professionals, insisted Butler, comprehended various processes and mechanisms of aging over the life course, from the cellular level to global contexts (Landrigan et al., 2005). Stated this way, the claim was consistent with his view that members of a geriatrics department would be the "essential colleague" in any medical school since aging is an essential component of the human life course.

Despite having other interests, Butler remained primarily concerned with geriatrics. He attributed difficulties in recruiting physicians to the field to persistent ageism in medicine, too little important research being done in gerontology, geriatrics' lack of prestige, and insufficient Medicare reimbursements for elder care. To remedy the situation, he pragmatically proposed (1) public-private partnerships to develop academic geriatric centers, (2) adjusting Medicare to cover current services and additional training, and (3) relating to medical students and residents the high satisfaction that geriatricians report (Beck & Butler, 2004).

"Intellectually and scientifically curious medical students need to be attracted to geriatrics," Butler reiterated in 2007, as if he were valorizing the pleasure he derived from being a clinician and a scientist. "There is glamour to research" (Butler, 2007). Regretting that Medicare and the Veterans Administration had cut the second year of geriatric fellowships, he contended that insufficient income was bound to diminish geriatrics and harm primary-care medicine (Karlin, Zeiss, & Burris, 2010). He concluded his plea on an angry note: "For physicians who ask, 'Why do we need geriatrics? I take care of plenty of older persons,' I would remind them that, although all their patients have hearts, this does not make them cardiologists" (Butler, 2007:2087; see also Bodenheimer, 2006:861–63; Woo, 2006).

Butler's work inspired academic medical centers around the country to build on research and clinical initiatives he had generated at Mount Sinai. He contributed to the creation of more than two dozen centers focused on research and training on Alzheimer's. His consultations with the John A.

Hartford and Donald Reynolds Foundations helped to reduce shortages of physicians, nurses, and social workers in the field of aging. Butler's colleagues and trainees spread his message (Bernard, Blanchette, & Brummel-Smith, 2009; Cassel, 2000; Hazzard, 2000; Libow, 2004). Despite cutbacks, ageism, and competing priorities within health centers, Butler tirelessly offered a vision of geriatrics that transcended intramural politics and financial shortfalls. His accomplishments are impressive.

Yet despite all his efforts, Butler never fully achieved his long-standing goal of creating a well-educated cadre of leaders to mentor those seeking to be trained to care for older people. Generalists and specialists, medical schools, and allied-health associations continue to struggle with the place of geriatrics in the health-care arena. Only thirty-three of ninety-eight specialties have requirements in geriatric medicine; conspicuously absent are general surgery and ophthalmology. Geriatric fellowships still go unfilled (von Preyss-Friedman, 2009).

In the most recent Institute of Medicine report (2008), thirty years after the initial one on aging and medicine, Chairman John Rowe and his colleagues noted that "while this population surge [the first boomers would turn sixty-five in 2011] has been foreseen for decades, little has been done to prepare the health care workforce for its arrival." Butler no doubt approved the institute's recommendation to define the geriatric workforce to include pharmacists, paraprofessionals (such as nurses' aides), caregivers, and patients. But he died wondering why Americans in and out of medical centers still resist taking sensible steps to address the visible consequences of population aging.

seven

RECASTING THE NEW GERONTOLOGY THROUGH THE INTERNATIONAL LONGEVITY CENTER

Chairing discussions about productive aging at the Salzburg Seminar in the early 1980s heightened Butler's sense that he and fellow idea brokers in gerontology should be addressing major aging-related issues on an international scale: "My own long-standing interest in the relationships among aging, productivity, and health was reinforced in no small measure by experiences gained during travels to different countries, Japan and the Soviet Union among them" (Butler & Gleason, 1985:xi–xii). Butler saw merit in inviting experts in the United States and abroad to meet to exchange strategies for tackling global issues such as income security, health promotion, and ageism.

The Salzburg Seminar enabled Butler to think outside the box about *productivity*, an issue of aging not yet central to researchers, educators, and practitioners. Reframing gerontological paradigms appealed to him. He liked to formulate new ways of thinking about growing older. But sometimes, he acknowledged, being a trailblazer could be a lonely, frustrating pursuit.

Butler had made his reputation as an expert on aging. He was first and foremost a physician and a scientist. Unfortunately this niche remained marginal (then and now) in the wider marketplace of ideas. Interest in ideas about age and aging (in contrast to theories of race, gender, and ethnicity) had not caught fire by 1980. Emerging scholars were entering the ranks of gerontologists and geriatricians, but other fields attracted many more newly minted professionals. Comparative approaches to gerontology, at first glance, frankly seemed an unpromising route for advancing research on aging. Except for occasional forays into the economics of retirement, health-care analyses, international affairs, policy studies, and anthropology, few U.S. investigators engaged in cross-cultural studies to address the varieties of aging. In pursuing critical issues in the context of global aging, Butler was ahead of his time.

In retrospect the Salzburg Seminar brought together some facets of Butler's formative years that would serve him well in maturity. He told me several times that his curiosity about foreign places began in youth. Wendell Willkie's *One World* (1943), a best-selling travelogue that pleaded for global peacekeeping, left a vivid impression. As a member of the U.S. Merchant Marine in World War II, Butler had traveled to several continents; he had worked while an undergraduate in Cuba as a purser for the Standard Fruit and Steamship Line. During the 1950s he avidly followed Jean Monnet's efforts to forge European unity. The gero-psychiatrist met leaders of the International Association of Gerontology in 1966 and attended a meeting in Austria.

STARTING THE INTERNATIONAL LONGEVITY CENTER

A 1987 trip to Japan boosted Butler's desire to create the first international partnership to promulgate fundamental principles, practices, and policies for aging societies (Butler & Kiikuni, 1993:xxiv). Prior to his visit, Sens. Alan Cranston and John Glenn and Rep. Claude Pepper had sent letters of introduction. Butler secured appointments with two prominent businessmen. One, Shigeo Morioka, the head of a major Japanese pharmaceutical firm, met with him on the day that the U.S. stock market lost 20 percent of its value. The men immediately thought that collaboration would be advantageous personally and strategically. Morioka became Butler's first partner in what became the International Longevity Center.

Thereafter Butler visited Japan several times a year, and he intently tracked two major developments. Japan was the country with the world's fastest growing older population; life expectancy at birth there had increased dramatically since World War II. The Japanese government's planning for the consequences of population aging, moreover, resulted in policies to transform work conditions, harness technology, and capitalize on the capacities of older workers ("Japan in the Year 2000," 1983; see also Ihara, ca. 1998). Over time Butler gained respect among Japan's elite. He was one of two speakers at a 1994 aging symposium sponsored by one of Japan's major newspapers. Butler recalled that the other speaker, Kenzaburō Ōe, who shortly thereafter won the Nobel Prize for Literature, spoke warmly of work done at Mount Sinai.

In 1990, with a seed grant from the oil company ARCO, Butler established the U.S. branch of the International Longevity Center (ILC-USA) at the Mount Sinai Medical Center to pursue policy issues related to the health and productivity of older persons. The center, according to Butler, was "to study the impact of population aging and advancing longevity from a socioeconomic perspective, health perspective, and quality of life" (Glaser, 2003; Mellan, 2010). That same year ILC-Japan was established under the directorship of Dr. Hideo Ibe.

The bilateral arrangement, with additional support from the Luce Foundation and the Japan Society, permitted Butler to arrange conferences to share lessons from Japanese experiences with people influential in policy making in North America. In his introduction to *Productive Aging and the Role of Older People in Japan* (1994:xiv), Butler identified four challenges or fears that people had related during his travels abroad. They were the very same anxieties he had heard expressed in the United States:

1. We cannot afford survival into late life.
2. Population aging will reduce our productive capacities.
3. An intergenerational crisis will emerge.
4. Older people might gain power that would be destructive to society.

To counteract pessimism and ageism, Butler commissioned empirical cross-cultural studies of population aging to highlight the personal and collective benefits of longevity as he and colleagues addressed various individual and societal impediments to realizing late-life potentials.

Butler became president and chief executive officer of ILC-USA in 1995. Though stepping down as chair of the Department of Geriatrics and Adult Development, he remained a professor of geriatrics at Mount Sinai Medical Center. ILC-USA gained tax-exempt status in 1998, which gave its board the right to independent governance. "For the ILC this is the best of both worlds," Butler remarked at the time. "We now have greater capacity to plan our own future while at the same time maintaining warm, familial ties with our parent organization" (ILC, 2011). A year later the International Longevity Center's operations moved to New York's Upper East Side; it took over a four-story, 8,000-square-foot building renovated by award-winning architect Richard Cook, who incorporated outside lighting and interior features to make the edifice safe, accessible, and eco-friendly.

All this came at a price. Renovations required considerable equity. Gifts from board members and friends, such as Laurence Rockefeller who contributed $250,000, alone would not sustain Butler's ambitious aims. ILC needed a predictable income flow to sponsor international exchanges. In addition the center typically had to contract for outside expertise to work on its projects. Butler failed in an attempt to tap trust funds from the Buck Foundation in California; fiscal scheming with entrepreneur Robert Gibson, while intellectually stimulating, did not bear fruit.

Luckily ILC-USA discovered a generous patron—or, more accurately, a "member patron" found Butler (Walker, 1991:198). Along with George Maddox (a Duke sociologist) and Janet Sainer (who had oversight for funding social services for older New Yorkers), Butler was invited to make a presentation to board members of Atlantic Philanthropies, then a low-key foundation and the brainchild of Charles Feeney, a cofounder of Duty-Free Shopping (LaMarche). Ray Handlan, the board chair, later invited Butler to flesh out big ideas for his International Longevity Center. By 2009 Atlantic Philanthropies had made grants totaling more than $5 billion. Over time Butler and ILC received in excess of $26 million (Butler, personal communication, January 2, 2010).

Atlantic Philanthropies encouraged Butler to build a network of experts to buttress ILC's work. Adept at forging partnerships at NIA and Mount Sinai, he approached organizations associated with the American Federation for Aging Research (which he had helped to establish) and ones that would give ILC access to resources in geriatrics medical education as well as develop ties with places such as the Fielding Graduate University, where Butler hoped to probe the relationship between wisdom and longevity (Butler, 1990). Such partnerships were deemed critical to advancing medical science at the end of the millennium. "This reliance on a complex network of experts in making health care policies mirrors the extent to which all that is entailed by 'modern medicine' has become arguably the single largest and most complex research-based technological system in the United States today" (Alliance Trends Resources, n.d.; American Federation for Aging, n.d.; Kraemer, 2006:179; Portal of Geriatric Online Education, n.d.).

ILC-USA advisers provided other useful contacts. That Butler could recruit influential, busy people attests to the ease with which he interacted with members of New York's various elites. On his board of directors were life-insurance executives, including Edward Berube, CEO of Futurity First Insurance Group, and Metropolitan Life's former CEO John J. Creedon; a nonprofit fundraiser, Naomi Levine, who successfully raised $2.5 billion for New York University; pharmaceutical executives such as Pfizer's Joe Feczko, MD, Paul Gilbert, cofounder of MedAvante, and Warner Lambert's Joseph Smith; two Nobel Laureates, biochemist Stanley Prusiner, MD, and economist Robert Fogel, whom Butler had funded at NIA; public officials, including Newark mayor Cory Booker as well as Senator and Mrs. John Glenn; powerful New York attorneys such as Lloyd Frank and William Zabel; financiers including Linda Lambert, a trustee of the Reynolds Foundation, and William Martin, cofounder of an online financial community; philanthropists, among them Evelyn Stefansson Nef, who served on Mount Sinai's board; and academic leaders such as Karen Hsu, Regina Peruggi (who once headed Marymount Manhattan College), and Catherine R. Simpson, dean of New York University's graduate school.

Butler also tapped the expertise of J. T. "Steve" Stephens, who launched a biotechnology firm; John Zweig, who headed global health-care marketing services; Lawrence Grossman, cochair of a public-interest initiative developing information technologies; and Humphrey Taylor, longtime chair of the Harris Poll. Among ILC's honorary board members were former senator Bill Bradley, First Lady Rosalynn Carter, television host Hugh Downs, Surgeon General C. Everett Koop, as well as Joshua Lederberg and Paul Marks, MD, respectively president emeriti of Rockefeller University and Memorial Sloan-Kettering Cancer Center.

On staff were trusted colleagues, many veterans of Butler's years at NIA or Mount Sinai. They included communications specialist Mal Schecter; friends such as gerontological social worker Rose Dobrof and Harry "Rick" Moody, a philosopher of aging with whom he had collaborated through Hunter College and the Brookdale Foundation; Barbara Paris, MD, whom he trained at Mount Sinai; as well as Larry D. Wright, MD, who directed the Schmieding Center for Senior Health; and University of Illinois-Chicago's S. Jay Olshansky, with whom Butler coauthored several important papers. Some staff members coordinated the various collaborative research projects under way. Others developed periodicals, special publications, websites, outreach programs, and a special Longevity Network. Butler, as always, made certain that he was accessible and responsive to the media.

International ties formed a third set of affiliations. Besides ILC-Japan's Shigeo Morioka, Butler greatly valued his counterparts in France, the United Kingdom, and the Dominican Republic. Francoise Forette, MD, an epidemiologist, dementia expert, and politician, arranged for him to speak at the French equivalent of the White House Conference on Aging, where he met President François Mitterand. Baroness Sally Greengross for many years headed Age Concern, which, like the National Council on the Aging, provides social services, job training and opportunities, information, and referrals. Rosy Pereyra worked with Julia Alvarez, the Dominican Republic's ambassador to the United States, to advocate for the aged in developing nations (Butler, personal communication, March 17, 2010). By 2009 seven other nations had established International Longevity Centers—Argentina, the Czech Republic, India, Israel, the Netherlands, Singapore, and South Africa. Negotiations were under way elsewhere when Butler died (ILC Global Alliance, 2009:ii).

Coordinating annual meetings at different international sites and engaging in ambitious, collaborative ventures with the dozen centers that constituted the ILC Global Alliance consumed much of Butler's time and effort. As he did at NIA and Mount Sinai Medical Center, Dr. Butler generated a daunting number of projects at the ILC (see "Decline," n.d.; "Tutoring," n.d.). To wit:

• With $12 million from Pfizer, three nations in the ILC network created an Alliance for Health & the Future, which explored how healthfulness and longevity contributed to increasing the wealth of countries. Drawing on United Nations resources, the ILC created a ninety-two-nation database to document the economic status of older people. Special attention was accorded to collecting data on job losses in later years in addition to information about women and minorities.

• With faculty from Columbia, NYU, and the State University of New York, the ILC conducted the World Cities Project to assess the health needs of older people in New York, London, Paris, and Tokyo. It also focused on the extent of old-age vulnerability in Newark, New Jersey. Besides investigating health disparities in metropolitan areas, the ILC instigated inquiries into emergency preparedness for older persons in post-9/11 New York, in Oklahoma City, and along the Gulf Coast after Hurricane Katrina.

• The ILC reached out to the media. The weeklong Age Boom Academy, founded in 2000 with seed funding from the New York Times Foundation, aimed over the course of the decade to deepen the understanding on the part of 150 journalists of how the perils and promises of societal aging affected their respective news beats. Ideas germinated in the academy often found mass circulation.

• ILC Scientific Conferences, often held at Canyon Ranch Health Resort near Tucson, Arizona, provided a useful forum for generating and disseminating basic and applied knowledge about aging. Topics ranged from cognition to sexuality. Butler told me that experts came pro bono to enjoy the amenities and intellectual stimulation. The conferences' success, in his opinion, reflected and sustained the "summoning power" of the International Longevity Center, helping to create a scientific basis for "the new gerontology" that had to take account of the latest developments in the biomedical and behavioral social sciences.

• ILC-USA, in collaboration with sister centers in Japan, France, the United Kingdom, and the Dominican Republic, proposed that a Declaration of the Rights of Older Persons be adopted at the second United National World Assembly on Ageing (2002). "At a time of misery and chaos for many older citizens of the world who have lost children and grandchildren in armed conflicts, who are often homeless and destitute, who suffer from malnutrition and ill health, and who live in societies that cannot provide them with basic necessities of life," Butler wished to stanch exploitation of and discrimination against older people. "We must not simply bear witness. We must compel change" (Butler, 2002a:152–53; see also Doron & Apter, 2010). Although the World Assembly did not adopt ILC proposal, Butler continued to seek to garner support for the declaration through publications and networks until he died.

LAYING THE FOUNDATION FOR THE
NEW GERONTOLOGY

A 1999 ILC scientific workshop attended by twenty-three participants and twenty-one observers heralded "the Promise of Basic Research on Aging . . . which could lead to biological interventions to prevent, delay, or reverse the adverse effects associated with aging, in particular the burden of disease." Butler's wide-ranging agenda at ILC built on priorities at NIA: (1) identifying genetic differences associated with life-span differences among species; (2) generating animal models to identify genes responsible for life-span extension and senescence; (3) determining linkages between DNA polymorphisms and longevity or age; (4) evaluating the role of oxidative damage in senescence; and (5) extending several decades of study on caloric reduction to prompt surrogate interventions to retard senescence without harming subjects (ILC, 1999:16, 19; see also Finch, 1994).

National Institute on Aging veteran Huber Warner affirmed the value of the ILC's strategy to review earlier NIA inquiries into basic biological mechanisms and processes of aging. Acknowledging that "normal" science proceeds incrementally, Warner counted on "a critical mass of investigators working in this area . . . because of NIA's efforts to stimulate research" (Warner, 2005:41). Butler encouraged investigators at the outset of every scientific International Longevity Center endeavor to update and assess relevant scientific findings; he was especially keen to identify diseases that would be generally accepted as "wake-up calls" if older people had better access to medical care and greater representation in clinical trials (Hayflick & Moody, 2003; ILC, 2000, 2002). Butler's decision to take inventory before moving forward was strongly endorsed by University of Michigan pathologist Richard A. Miller, MD, PhD. A frequent ILC participant, Miller identified three lines of evidence worth exploring:

> One genetic, one based on dietary restriction, and one phylogenetic—lead to an important conclusion: although the signs of aging are, to a first approximation, similar in all species of mammals, the pace at which these changes can be coordinately regulated and, in some cases, by as simple a change as the modification of a single base of DNA sequence or the restriction of food availability. Fifty years ago an assertion that the rate of aging might be deliberately modified would have been only a hunch or statement of faith, without empirical foundation. Today, however, it is clear that the rate of aging can differ among members of the same species and differ radically between species as closely related as monkeys and people.
>
> (MILLER, 2002:163–64)

Miller's prospectus helped to set into motion objectives for necessary scientific research under the aegis of the International Longevity Center.

Revisiting age-related knowledge in this manner proved to have profound implications in laying the foundations for what Butler early on envisioned to be "the New Gerontology" (1983c:351). Among other things, Butler and his teams of researchers recognized issues unresolved in previous scientific endeavors. Should medical scientists and public-health researchers study more than one disease at a time? What obstacles (political and ethical as well as scientific) limit maximizing longevity? In what ways would extra years turn out to be both a gift and a bane? Such research questions (and others) emboldened Butler to envision interdisciplinary scientific explorations beyond those on which he had embarked either at NIA or at Mount Sinai.

For example, Butler postulated that genetic factors accounted for 30 percent of the rate of human aging and life expectancy; environmental and behavioral factors explained the rest of the risk factors. His hypotheses about the genetic basis of aging were grounded on developments still being assessed in research laboratories during the past decade. In the case of studies of fruit flies, Butler reported, "scientists have identified a variety of single gene mutations that either increase their life expectancy or modify the extension of life expectancy by other mutations" (2003a). He speculated that genes that reduced early-life pathology might not reveal much to scientists about aging and senescence.

At the same time newly available scientific insights dissuaded Butler from proposing human genetic manipulation. Unconvinced that findings obtained from studying primitive organisms could be extrapolated very far to humans, Butler recast familiar gerontological principles—ones evident in the 1963 NIMH report, *Human Aging*—into a new research strategy.

> The ultimate payoff for this genetic research is to learn enough about aging to identify promising avenues for nongenetic interventions to delay, prevent, or even reverse the adverse age-related changes leading to disease and disability in humans. . . . It is important to note that the goal of these studies is not to find ways of altering human genes but to learn enough about aging to extend years of active healthy life without genetic alteration.
>
> (2003a:20; cf. WARNER ET AL., 1987:22–23, 30)

That Butler wanted to redirect aging research on evolutionary, not genetic, grounds illustrates his willingness to meld experience and critical thinking as he assessed pathways most likely to advance gerontology as a science.

Other strands of scientific information seemed to justify placing high on the aging research agenda the revision and elaboration of evolutionary theories. Butler cited observational data, biostatistics, correlations between longevity and skeletal maturation, the declining function of vital organs, and investigations into the lives of cells. "We haven't found any biologic reason not to live to 110," Butler concluded. "I'll go a bit further. It is my best estimate that our biogenetic maximum life span is 120 years—approximately 1 million hours" (Bortz, 2007:5–6). He illustrated his judgment about the maximum length of the human life span fancifully in a coauthored article in *Scientific American:* humans designed for healthy lives as centenarians, he claimed, would have bigger ears, curved necks, extra padding around joints, and shorter limbs (Olshansky, Carnes, & Butler, 2003).

It is important to note that Butler wished to ensure the advancement of research on aging by grounding it in the latest biomedical investigations. Scientists, he contended, must expand previous studies of caloric reduction, biomarkers, mammalian models, and comparative studies of biological mechanisms. Recent discoveries, however, had prompted new lines of scientific inquiry worth pursuing, such as breakthroughs that explored the efficacy of environmental and behavioral factors such as exercise on human performance. Butler also endorsed translational research that should eventuate in successful drug interventions (Brekke, Eli, & Palinkas, 2007; Satterfeld et al., 2009; Woolf, 2008).

On strategic grounds Butler understood that he faced resistance to proposing that longevity studies be conducted under the gerontological canopy. Over the years he had seen ageism among health professionals undercut the impact of research on age and aging. Now, he anticipated, many colleagues in geriatrics and gerontology (to defend principles and to protect vested interests) probably would criticize any initiative that aimed at adding years in late life. "No one who speaks in public about longevity research goes very far before encountering the widespread belief that research on extending the life span is unethical," observed Richard Miller (2002:170). "It also does little good to point out that a similar argument could have been made 200 years ago against penicillin, plumbing systems, and surgical anesthesia." To collaborators at ILC, mapping out a new paradigm was worth the risk.

The greatest threat, Butler felt, came from advocates of anti-aging programs, who gained adherents and customers for their promises that their interventions could eradicate senescence, thereby making immortality possible. In Butler's opinion, science did not warrant the claims made by proponents of anti-aging medicine. To be credible, the possibility of extending the human life span had to be validated by human biomarkers, which ILC research partners repeatedly declared did not yet exist. Worse, in an opinion he repeatedly stated, the anti-aging coalition guaranteed positive results from interventions (such as diet pills and hormone replacements), which lacked approval from the U.S. Food and Drug Administration. Many "natural drugs" had been shown in fact to cause adverse reactions (Butler, 2003; see also ILC, 2002; Warner, 2005:1006–8).

Which scientific community did lay audiences actually think spoke the truth about aging? Most people lacked the necessary knowledge to base a decision on scientific grounds, but they surely would take note of the sizes of respective constituent members. Advocates of anti-aging medicine hugely outnumbered gerontologists. With greater resources for advertising and access to media outlets, the American Academy of Anti-Aging Medicine, whose members ranged from well-meaning researchers to outright charlatans, succeeded in undercutting the value of gerontologic and geriatric investigations and trumpeting their own claims (Binstock, 2003; Haber, 1974; Leslie, 1974).

Meanwhile researchers on aging like Butler were tracking another disturbing trend: unless their habits changed, boomers were likely to be the first cohort in recent U.S. history to be less healthy than their parents. Steady gains in life expectancy that the United States had enjoyed for decades seemed unlikely to continue, in part because Americans were eating more and exercising less. The prevalence of obesity, which had increased by roughly 50 percent per decade in the 1980s and 1990s, had a substantially negative effect on longevity. Another factor contributing to diminished life expectancy in the United States was the increase in infectious diseases. Also significant were widening health disparities prevalent among men from minority and ethnic groups in terms of strokes, heart problems, and work-related disabilities (Olshansky et al., 2005; Olshansky, 2009).

Despite real obstacles to continuing gains in life expectancy, Butler, true to form, presented the case for longevity research in optimistic terms. He rebuked those who argued that aging populations threatened societal well-being. "I think that these social pessimists are forgetting that the new longevity and the aging of our population are reflections of . . . social, techno-logical, and economic success. Longevity is a blessing," he proclaimed. "This longevity revolution is a scion of the industrial revolution. Better nutrition, improved sanitation, higher standards of living, socioeconomic progress— all account for this new longevity" (Butler & Kiikuni, 1993:xxiii, 169).

That humans could enjoy an extra number of healthful, productive years resulted from a combination of demographic and dietary factors, advances in public health and medicine, as well as historically driven socio-economic vectors. "Behind the broad changes," noted Butler, going a step further, were "*ideas*, and *ideas* spur changes" (Butler & Kiikuni, 1993:xxiii).

Widely held reservations, indeed fears, about longevity's promises did not abate, however. People questioned how beneficial it might be to have elders gain additional years of life. Accordingly, even optimists like Butler had to temper their enthusiasm:

> Despite this great achievement of widespread longevity, there are many fears that haunt societies. One is the fear that somehow the increasing number and proportion of older persons in the population may lead to economic stagnation and may impose a greater burden upon our societies than they can reasonably withstand. There are also fears that the rapid aging of populations will lead to intergenerational conflict. We must address these fears and recognize that longevity has always been a relative concept.
>
> (BUTLER & KIIKUNI, 1993:XX–XXI)

Little could be done immediately to allay such fears. Revolutionary ideas, such as productively harnessing global gains in longevity, would take root slowly. "Both the industrial-scientific revolution, now about 200 years old, and the longevity revolution, less than 100 years old, have occurred with great rapidity," Butler observed. "It will take time to complete adaptations to the longevity revolution which will require imagination, skill, and the fair distribution of resources" (Butler & Jasmin, 2000:20).

Talking about longevity (with or without explicit reference to age and aging) fomented its own set of conundrums. Short-term politics and self-serving politicians, as Maggie Kuhn had pointed out, would undermine longevity ideals—or, for that matter, long-term policy goals in general (Butler & Kiikuni, 1993:102). And as Myrna Lewis noted, attention needed to be paid to gender disparities, which would grow more pernicious as societies aged. Women, who on average outlive men, often lack resources in later years as health problems mount. Accordingly, Lewis recommended that savings and other money be set aside in women's names, and that women organize for mutual support. In 2003 Lewis created the first women's longevity group under her direction as a psychotherapist. Other professional groups and informal gatherings met, led by women to facilitate discussions (ILC, 2003; Lewis, 2005:1–2).

Butler wanted longevity science to feed into research on gerontology. To him it was partly a matter of refocusing issues. His tack paralleled the approach to age enunciated by Nobel laureate Elie Wiesel: "Everyone is trying to grow old without looking old. . . . No one likes old age now; it's called longevity; that sounds better" (Butler & Jasmin, 2000:283). Yet name changes, even ones more than cosmetic, would not put into motion a paradigm shift. To actualize the new gerontology demanded a new level of cross-disciplinary synergy. "The full realization of the opportunities resulting from the longevity revolution will depend on many actions that are, in principle, within our control. They are within our control as individuals and as family members. They are within our control as workers, professionals, scientists, leaders in civic, healthcare, and nonprofit institutions," declared Harvey V. Fineberg, a policy expert at the Harvard School of Public Health. "The deeper and lasting challenge of the worldwide revolution in longevity" demanded scientific ingenuity, personal discipline, collective responsibility, and political courage sufficient "to seize the opportunity that the longevity revolution represents and leverage that opportunity into a reality of a more successful society" (Butler & Jasmin, 2000:289).

In fact, legitimating longevity science entailed redrawing gerontology's boundaries. In *Longevity and the Quality of Life* (2000), Butler indicated that the longevity revolution swept conceptually from cellular and molecular biology to biomedical and behavioral strategies for rearranging institutions. It focused on individual, familial, and societal needs and responsibilities for providing education, health promotion, and disease prevention. "Society has experienced many positive developments [which] has led people to plan even more for the future," he affirmed. "The aging revolution is also contributing to a transformation of our health care and service delivery systems by requiring a more comprehensive, integrated approach to patient care, by the development of new technology to deal more effectively than we presently do with the frail and bedridden, and by advancing long-term care programs for all ages and conditions, including decisions about palliative and end-of-life care" (Butler & Jasmin, 2000:20; see also Keene, 2008).

In presenting his vision of the new gerontology, Butler was making a profound contribution to the literature on longevity science. Of the many immediate consequences of the Longevity Revolution, he opined, the "least noted has been the extent to which health and longevity have enhanced the prospects of greater riches, of the material kind" (2005a:551). To accentuate the originality of his line of reasoning, Butler reintroduced the concept of "failures of success," which he first borrowed from Ernest Gruenberg in the 1970s. (Gruenberg hypothesized that medical progress often spawns unexpected and negative consequences.) The rise of failures of success, reasoned Butler, helped to explain the grip on popular and scientific thinking of ageist assumptions concerning societal aging.

Since the 1980s naysayers had warned that growing numbers of sick, dependent elders would burden younger people with an "aging crisis." A zero-sum war for limited resources would ensue. Butler denounced as ageist neoconservative proposals to avert generational conflict by reducing public pensions and containing the rate of growth of health-care costs:

> If the growth of ageing populations and advancing longevity are indeed "failures of success"—the uncontrollable and unfortunate by-products of

social-economic and medical progress—then it stands to reason that fundamental and clinical biomedical research should be halted. The medical and
other helping professions as well as research institutions should instead direct their resources and imagination solely to marginal repairs of mental and
physical disorders and to cost savings.

(2005a:547)

Butler's competing model optimistically invoked the "Longevity Dividend." The extension of healthy lives not only generates wealth for individuals but also bolsters the political economy. Conversely, he argued, the
compression of morbidity and mortality rates would afford aging populations more productive years to contribute to societal well-being. If scientists could slow aging by seven years, the age-specific risk of frailty, disability, and death would be reduced by approximately half at every age. And
that should result, Butler reasoned, in shorter periods during which rising
generations of elders would rely on age-based entitlements and health-care
programs. "The science of aging has the potential to produce what we refer
to as a 'Longevity Dividend' in the form of social, economic, and health
bonuses both for individuals and entire populations—a dividend that
would begin with generations currently alive and continue for all that follow" (Olshansky, Miller, & Butler, 2006:31–32).

Knowing that he had ventured with little training into relatively un-
charted areas of the social sciences, Butler sought independent validation
of the economics of the Longevity Dividend. Initially he was disheartened
by expert opinions. James P. Smith, a senior economist at RAND, argued
in 1999 that "the relation between better health and more wealth or larger
changes in wealth . . . is uninformative about causality." Three years later,
however, William Nordhaus, a Yale professor associated with the National
Bureau of Economic Research, argued that "improvements in health status
have been a major contributor to economic welfare over the twentieth century." In fact, Nordhaus contended, "the economic values of increases in
longevity . . . [and] the medical revolution over the last century appears to
qualify, at least from an economic point of view, for Samuel Johnson's ac-
colade as 'the greatest benefit to mankind' " (2002:37–38).

Additional support soon was forthcoming. Anthony Webb, an economist at ILC-USA, produced an Alliance Policy Report, *Do Health and Longevity Create Wealth?* (2006). Literally taking to heart Virgil's aphorism, which declared that "Health is the greatest wealth," Webb contended that "increases in longevity are associated with improvements in the average level of health, particularly among older persons." Based on studies of household behavior and macrolevel cross-cultural studies, he concluded that "the emerging evidence is that health is really fundamental to worker productivity and stimulates the investments in physical and human capital that are essential to economic growth" (2006:21–22; see also Marmot, 2006; Pan, Chai, & Farber, 2007).

THE LONGEVITY REVOLUTION

The Longevity Revolution: The Benefits and Challenges of Living a Long Life (2008; hereafter *TLR*) was published when Robert Butler, at age eighty-one, was being acclaimed in the United States and abroad as a vigorous and astute elder of the tribe. Fifteen years in the making, *TLR* appeared more than three decades after *Why Survive? Being Old in America*. (Butler had written his Pulitzer Prize winner in his late forties, when he was not yet widely known among gerontologists.) *Why Survive?* and *The Longevity Revolution* synthesize the research and ideas of many colleagues in the field. Whereas *Why Survive?* sparked the imaginations of experts and informed citizens by filling a void, *TLR* did not live up to expectations in terms of sales or impact.

Butler had a reputation for writing provocatively, couching arguments in dense data. *Why Survive?* was didactic and angry. It sought to catalog and excoriate the myriad obstacles created by interactions and institutions that hindered people from enjoying fulfilling lives in later years. In contrast, *TLR* sounded a more optimistic note:

> With the Longevity Revolution, the world enters a new and unprecedented stage of human development—the impact of which has been made greater because of its rapidity. We are no longer limited to a life view that must

accommodate itself to the historic brevity of life, to random and premature illness and death, as Thomas Hobbes described it. The Longevity Revolution is a great intellectual and social as well as medical achievement and an opportunity that demands changes in outmoded mind-sets, attitudes, and socioeconomic arrangements. Many of our economic, political, ethical, health and other institutions, such as education and work life, have been *rendered obsolete* by the added years of life for so many citizens. The social construct of old age, even the inner life and activities of older persons, is now subject to a positive revision.

(17)

Butler's underlying premise is that the Longevity Revolution represents the latest transformation in the history of humankind: "Health, longevity, and aging engender wealth" (27). *TLR*'s thesis, which relied primarily on work commissioned through the International Longevity Center, stipulates two themes. First, longer-lived individuals should be grateful to have control and responsibility for their lives (98). Second, extra years should impel elders to make meaningful contributions to others, which in turn would promote harmony across generations (397).

As he had stressed in *Why Survive?*, Butler considered ageism chief among the obstacles that denied individuals the benefits of attaining late life. In *TLR* he goes a step further and conflates ageism with *gerontophobia*, that is, a fear of growing old:

> The underlying basis of ageism is the dread and fear of growing older, becoming ill and dependent, and approaching death. People are afraid, and that leads to profound ambivalence. The young dread aging, and the old envy youth. Behind ageism is corrosive narcissism, the inability to accept our fate, for indeed we are all in love with our youthful selves, as is reflected in the yearning behind the expression "salad days." Although undoubtedly universal, ageism in the United States is probably fueled by the worship of youth in a still-young country dominated by the myth of the unending frontier. . . . *Denial is a close cousin of ageism; in effect, it eliminates aging from consciousness.*

(44–45)

Butler claims in *TLR* that ageism extends from inner consciousness to cultural archetypes: "Beyond concerns about maintaining productivity, we must address the underlying terror and distaste for aging, replete as it is with hysteria and anger, which ultimately becomes a self-afflicting prejudice" (29). He diagnoses ageism as a "psychosocial disease." Treating and eradicating ageism would require legislative initiatives and different cultural sensibilities. The urgency mounts, he emphasizes: "We all chance to become its ultimate victims as longevity increases" (53).

The significance of the paradigm shift occasioned by the Longevity Revolution, argues Butler, demands radical and global changes in conventional frames of reference and long-standing ways of speaking. "Human interest in longevity is not always the same as the love of life. Some are simply greedy for an extended life but have no capacity to enjoy it. And those with a passion for life may be heedless about its perpetuity," he observes (103). Ageism, in fact, fuels "the three great fears of longevity—that there will be an unprecedented number of economically dependent older persons, that old people will drag down economic productivity, and that there will be intergenerational conflict" (255). Adding to this trio of horrors, he reminds readers that "Alzheimer's disease is a disorder of longevity," along with Parkinson's disease and amyotrophic lateral sclerosis (Lou Gehrig's disease) (127, 132). With added longevity comes the threat of frailty and loss of autonomy.

To grapple with the various physical, psychological, and social forces that limit individuals' opportunities to partake of longevity's fruits, Butler invokes remedies that he had been advancing for decades. He appeals for (1) increases in government spending, especially at the National Institutes of Health, earmarked for basic biological studies into how we age and live long, (2) disease-targeted research, and (3) improved lifestyles that would enhance healthy, productive aging (119, 162). Relying on resources in the private sector, he felt, simply would not suffice. Butler simultaneously insists that the scope of geriatrics be enlarged to provide comprehensive care along a continuum from preventive medicine, through health promotion, to end-of-life care. He implores older Americans to stay active by engaging in voluntary assistance to families in need, performing community service, and doing unpaid mentoring in schools (242–43).

To enhance chances for success in reaping the benefits of the Longevity Revolution, declares Butler, scientific investigators have to embrace the New Gerontology. It is time to move beyond a recapitulation of the myths and stereotypes about aging that had inspired researchers associated with the Duke Longitudinal Studies and the NIMH study of *Healthy Aging* in the 1950s. Nor is it enough to concentrate scientific efforts on understanding of underlying mechanisms of aging or to intensifying the search for causes of diseases prevalent in later years. "The most important aspect of the new gerontology is the introduction of preventive, therapeutic, and rehabilitative interventions, which include social and behavioral strategies," Butler asserts. *"Research is both the ultimate cost containment and the ultimate human resource"* (182–84). In so doing, he amplifies a dictum by Lewis Thomas (1999): "I do not believe that looking for new information about nature, at whatever level, can possibly be called unnatural."

A fresh set of research strategies follows from conceiving of age and aging under the umbrella of the New Gerontology. According to Butler, regenerative medicine and genomics can become powerful treatments in delaying the onset and progression of various diseases. If biomedical researchers can figure out a way to delay the occurrence of Alzheimer's by as little as five years, he claims, the incidence of this scourge can be cut in half. Postponing dependency among persons over sixty-five for one month would save $5 billion per month (in 1993 dollars) (184). More radically, Butler calls for a revolutionary approach to biomedical research that inevitably would undercut the raison d'être of the National Institutes of Health: "The historic biomedical research approach has been largely devoted to the study of one disease at a time, as if each was totally independent of the other, whereas underlying all diseases is the reality of aging. It is therefore time to supplement the disease-by-disease research approach by providing new intellectual and material resources dedicated to the underlying biology that predisposes us all to disease, disability, and ultimately death" (185). He acknowledges that the paradigm shift will be costly. "The present level of development of aging and longevity research justifies an Apollo-type effort to control aging, extend the healthy life, and equalize life expectancies adversely affected by socioeconomic class, gender, ethnicity, and race" (187). The allusion to the nation's success in space is intentional. Butler characterized John Glenn's return flight in space at age seventy-six as an American hero's effort to seek new frontiers for older Americans. His friend's courage afforded scientists insights into the effects of antigravity on sleep and organ systems among the healthy aged. Such explorations, however costly, seemed worthwhile (Butler, 1998a; see also "Space Aging," 1998).

The price tag for Butler's big dreams nonetheless seemed astronomical even to his likely supporters. Over the course of his career, U.S. presidents such as Richard Nixon, Ronald Reagan, and George W. Bush had steadily undermined the liberal agenda for health, education, and welfare enunciated by leaders from Franklin Delano Roosevelt through Lyndon Baines Johnson. By the beginning of the new millennium, neoconservative lawmakers at the federal and state levels had grown bolder session after session in their attempts to contain the growth of social and health services. Aware that he was out of sync, Butler had to figure out ways to make the short-term costs of his agenda palatable and manageable. He anticipated that policy makers would have to redesign Medicaid and Medicare and modify Social Security.

Not all savings had to result from cutbacks. As in the past, Butler felt that investing in research was cost effective, albeit sometimes in serendipitous ways. He urges scientists to seize on medical principles and practices consonant with the inexorable needs of an aging society. He also insists that taking effective steps hinged on the willingness of scientific communities to reorder interdisciplinary priorities, however incrementally. "Eventually, two academic, scientifically based specialties will emerge and possibly merge," he forecasts. There will be *a longevity-oriented medicine*, concerned with preserving and promoting health and longevity, and *geriatrics*, which will deal with both the assessment and coordination of care of those who are impaired. It will be dedicated to the restoration and rehabilitation of functions, and the struggle against frailty and dependency" (2008:220).

Having identified "the health politics of anguish" at NIH and having been bruised in mean turf battles at Mount Sinai, Butler recognized the dangers in designating "the politics of longevity" as the thematic and strategic linchpin for the New Gerontology. To galvanize support for his ideas across the age spectrum, he insists that researchers on aging probe continuities and changes over the life course to order to gauge the range of conditions and sensibilities in late life. Gerontologists should not just recruit subjects over age sixty-five; they also need younger subjects. As he proceeds, Butler recalls heated debates with his friend the late Senator Cranston from California. Cranston believed that "biomedical research will soon increase not only life expectancy but life span"—a position that Butler rejects on scientific grounds (314). He knows that the so-called longevity lobby complicates the politics of aging: "It is important to differentiate for those key decision makers that the goal of gerontology is to extend the prime years of life, not length of life per se," he insists. "On balance, the more intense members of the longevity lobby have unwittingly held back the development of gerontology" (314–15).

The Longevity Revolution is a tour de force. Its insights reflect experiences over more than a half-century of thinking. Here, toward the end of his life, Butler challenges himself and others to redirect science and to reorient policies so that humans can live their lives in healthful, fruitful, meaningful ways. Many reviewers agreed. USC biologist Caleb Finch (2009) claimed that "with its magisterial synthesis and penetrating insights over a dazzling range, the *Longevity Revolution* belongs on the short shelf of great writings that have guided the public debates on aging for policymakers and for informing the public on tangible goals ahead." Leonid Gavrilov and Natalia Gavrilova (2008), writing from the Center on Aging at the University of Chicago, described the book as "unique in that Butler not only describes the medical and social problems that can be anticipated when baby boomers reach retirement age but also suggests bold and radical solutions for these upcoming problems." Some qualified their praise. A. Mark Clarfield, MD, a geriatrician at Ben Gurion University in Israel, felt that in one section "the author goes off the track to discuss how to overcome far-reaching problems such as famine, war, pestilence as well as a potpourri of other topics." Nonetheless, Clarfield went on to stay that "when this man writes a new book, US physicians should take notice" (2009:107–8).

Not surprisingly, it was Butler's claim that the Longevity Revolution is as significant as other seismic societal shifts (such as the Civil Rights movement, the feminist revolution, or global warming) that caused some readers discomfort. He dares to stake a claim for a vision that extends far beyond the customary niche for gerontologists and geriatricians. For those accustomed to marginalizing research on aging, *TLR* was too audacious, too strident in its bid to move the field to center stage. It fell victim to its bold, often complex, orthogonal presentation—precisely the sort of forward-looking, cross-disciplinary way of thinking that, ironically, once had brought Butler to the forefront of his field. In any event, *TLR*'s prescriptions for altering health services and investing more heavily in research on aging never really had a chance of enactment in an era of fiscal austerity.

Butler himself was disappointed that *TLR* did not have greater impact. He had hoped for another best seller that prompted critical analysis and corrective action. When it did not happen, he told me that he understood why. Publishing houses in recent years had issued thousands of books on aging that promised readers, with little evidence, that they never needed to grow old. *TLR* offered neither nostrums nor conventional wisdom nor quick fixes. Books by friends—Gene Cohen's *The Mature Mind* and Marc Freedman's *Encore*—were better written. Consequently, *The Longevity Revolution* faced greater competition for sales, novelty, and influence than had *Why Survive?* (Bennett, 2011).

More issues than lower-than-anticipated book sales were consuming Butler, however. Sickness and death preoccupied him while he was preparing the final drafts of *The Longevity Revolution*. A reversal of fortunes shadowed his life until he died. Since trying times in childhood and adulthood, he had somehow managed to convey an upbeat message and optimistic tone; he chose to get on with business precisely the way that he encouraged others to do. If he were to affirm life's promises and prospects, as was his custom, he had to refuse to settle for mere survival. But family, friends, and fame could not inure him to tragedy.

A SEASON OF GRIEF AND SADNESS

Since Myrna Lewis was a very healthy sixty-seven-year-old, the couple first attributed her uncharacteristic sluggishness in 2005 to jetlag after a long trip. But fatigue per se could not explain a disturbing set of symptoms that persuaded her to present herself at Mount Sinai Medical Center that June. There she was diagnosed with glioblastima multiforme. For a while the tumor shrunk, but by mid-September her health was deteriorating. Her husband, four children, a grandchild, and her home health aide were by Myrna's bedside in her home when she died early in the morning of November 15, 2005. "It was devastating," Butler told Claudia Dreifus, a *New York Times* reporter, a year later. "I haven't recovered." He added, "One of the many ways Myrna's death affects me is that we can't reminisce together. But it's worse than that; there is just this terrific loneliness. You keep going. Being left alone is one of the facts of aging. There's data that suggests that people can actually die of a broken heart, become sick because of it" (Dreifus, 2006). Butler grieved for Myrna Lewis until he died. Together they had shared love, family, travel, writing, and high adventures. But Butler kept on going, sometimes entering into relationships with strong women. His relationship with Barbara Walters ("Does Barbara Walters"; "Barbara Walters") was public knowledge. During his last year of life, Butler became close to Herta Gordon, an Austrian-born sculptress.

Butler's professional commitments did not taper off after Lewis died. He traveled, granted interviews, and interacted with gerontologists and geriatricians. He delighted in learning new ideas, meeting new people. Never giving a thought to retirement, he had a multiyear plan for books to write, lectures to give, and important work remaining to do.

Much to his dismay, Butler discovered that ensuring the future of the International Longevity Center had to become a major concern of his. The recession of 2008 crippled the ILC. Even before the economic downturn, Butler lost significant support from Atlantic Philanthropies, which was dedicated to spending down its assets and going out of business. "I am indebted to Dr. Robert Butler for building my consciousness about aging issues," declared Gara LaMarche at the 2007 annual meeting of Grantmakers in Aging. Without publicly stating that the Philanthropies had other priorities, LaMarche noted that the number of foundations "which ought to be concerned with aging is almost infinite." (LaMarche, 2011a, 2011b; Proscio, 2010).   Unfortunately the times were not auspicious for another "member patron" to rescue the ILC.

This left Butler three options: He could disband the International Longevity Center. He could negotiate new terms of affiliation with Mount Sinai Medical Center, which seemed unlikely given his strained relations with Mount Sinai's president and new chair of Geriatrics and Palliative Care. Butler determined that his best course of action was to make arrangements with Columbia University, where he had friends in Public Health, Social Work, and elsewhere on campus. The prospect of returning to his alma mater, with its formidable strengths in international affairs and his beloved Core Curriculum, made him happy.

eight

AMERICA'S AGING VISIONARY

At age seventy-nine, Butler reported in 2006 that he had started to take better care of his physical health after his wife Myrna died:

> Since her death, I've been very protective of myself, quite purposively. I go to bed earlier. I've been more thoughtful about my diet and activity levels. I pace myself. On weekends, I have this walking club. A whole group of us walk six miles through the city. I feel like I have to take care of myself. I still have work to do. And it's important work!
>
> (DREIFUS, 2006)

Robert Butler always enjoyed very good health, notwithstanding a bout in childhood with scarlet fever and recurring insomnia that had first afflicted him early in his medical practice. Only those who knew him well would have thought that they noticed any signs of decline.

Surgery after a gall bladder attack in 2008, Butler acknowledged, caused him to feel a bit frail. He walked more carefully thereafter, but he still exercised regularly. Walking was the sort of cardiovascular exercise that

Butler recommended to older people. He routinely gave friends and ac-
quaintances Digi-Walkers, with the International Longevity Center logo,
to encourage them to walk at least five thousand paces per day.

Work remained paramount, as it had all his life. Butler's diaries indicate
that he was logging sixty-hour weeks up until he died (Butler, personal
communication, March 2010). Drawing inspiration from the nation's rising
number of centenarians, he expected himself to reap additional dividends
from living a long, fruitful life. "The older you live, the healthier you have
been," he declared. Most centenarians "didn't smoke, they didn't drink ex-
cessively, they have personal relationships that are pretty darn good, they
have a sense of humor, they care about life and what life offers and
they have a sense of purpose" (George, 2010).

Butler's own attitudes toward growing older had not changed much as
he advanced in years. He told me that he did not really start to feel old
until his mother died in 1993, when he was sixty-six; professionally he
sometimes felt that he fell prey to age discrimination. That said, Butler
lived the productive, healthy lifestyle in old age that he prescribed for others. He treasured "the preciousness of life and especially the great importance of family. I am a father of four wonderful daughters who remain loyal
in both practical and loving ways" (Bensing, 2008). Recent surveys conducted by the National Council on the Aging and Harris Interactive, moreover, confirmed his impression that Americans' perceptions about aging
were moving in a positive direction. "Respondents view older persons as
younger than they did only 25 years ago," Butler (2008) noted. A *New
Yorker* cartoon heralding seventy as the new fifty pleased him, for it underscored that "this [shift] is associated with a decline in both physical and
mental disability rates."

Butler shared practical insights about healthful aging in his final book,
The Longevity Prescription (2010a). His aim was "to use the accumulated
knowledge, research, and resources of the International Longevity Center
(ILC) in order to offer [readers] the best strategies to live long *and* to live
well" (1). Promising neither magic pills nor elixirs, *The Longevity Prescription* did spell out efficacious ways for aging well. He felt that an understanding of longevity science could differentiate beneficial from deleteri-

ous lifestyles; persons of any age could and should select appropriate strategies for healthy living. *The Longevity Prescription* offered nine scripts. At least half the formulas prescribed positive outlooks and connections with others: (1) maintain mental vitality, (2) nurture your relationships, (3) seek essential sleep, (4) set stress aside, (5) connect with your community, (6) live the active life, (7) eat your way to health, (8) practice prevention, and (9) stay with the strategy. "The goal, boldly stated, is to be happier, healthier, and more at ease with yourself" (263).

There were times, Butler admitted, when he found it difficult to follow his own recommendations, "to do things that rouse the quiet stream of happiness that you know is there" (264). He grew more and more disturbed by the ugly side of U.S. history as the presidency of George W. Bush unfolded. In discussions he repeatedly surprised me with unexpected denunciations of slavery and Indian massacres during the colonial era; these dark moments presaged a horrible pattern that (according to Butler) continued through the nation's support of dictators and indifference to revelations of genocide abroad. The dreadful saga, he declaimed, extended into the present day. A man who had been circumspect about his politics in public, Butler in private did not hesitate to bemoan widening disparities in wealth, a succession of poor domestic leadership, a skein of misbegotten foreign policies, as well as an unfathomable waste of human capital and environmental resources. As a result of misguided actions past and present, Butler— showing flashes of anger and shock over the pattern of folly and deceit— declared that America was forsaking its democratic promises as it squandered opportunities for transformations that had seemed attainable earlier in his life. Now in his eighties, he began to feel ideologically and politically marginalized.

In addition, Butler admitted to me that personal disappointments engendered some of his disillusionment. Whereas the graying of America could have been an impetus for giving higher priority to old-age policy making, aging issues still had little traction in Washington. He was furious that Congress voted only modest budget increases to the National Institute on Aging. Allocations to NIA remained far less than Congress authorized for doing cancer research or seeking cures for heart ailments and infectious diseases (Sheets, Bradley, & Hendricks, 2006:51). Even friends in Congress were unreceptive to Butler's idea that 1 percent of the Medicare budget should be earmarked to underwrite gerontological research. Owing to economic woes at the beginning of the millennium, U.S. lawmakers were disinclined to provide the resources, financial and otherwise, that Butler thought were needed to support NIA researchers who investigated mechanisms and processes of aging and sought to develop technological and pharmacological interventions.

Nor did health-care educators implement Butler's recommendations to revamp medical training, as much as he had hoped. Experts agreed that there were not enough providers trained in geriatrics to care for baby boomers. Yet the gap between professionals and patients could not be bridged. Fellowships that Butler had decades earlier created at NIA went unfilled in a new millennium. Also languishing were research and clinical training opportunities that private foundations funded on his recommendation. Chairs of departments of internal medicine, surgery and other specialties continued to claim (over Butler's objections) that they had requisite on-hand expertise in gerontology and geriatrics. To justify their conviction, they pointed to successful experiences in treating older patients in waiting rooms and hospital beds. Yet the aged rarely received adequate treatment for depression or other mental illnesses, substance abuse or sexually transmitted diseases. No wonder Butler considered ageism rampant in medical settings.

The aging of baby boomers did not improve notions about (old) age in the United States; ageism remained virulent. Biases festered throughout American society, from faith-based communities to fitness centers. Computer literacy and social networking came more easily to Generation X than to boomers. Older actors considered themselves lucky to find small parts in movies and television. Snickers and silence about what to expect in late life reinforced prejudices and fears about growing older, despite uncertainties in youth and adulthood. Age discrimination eroded many older people's sense of worth and identity. Ageism fanned dread across generations, disturbing successive cohorts about their future selves.

Concerns about societal aging added to the woes of individual aging. Many pundits portrayed an ominous picture of age-based class warfare in the making. They contrasted the debts of underemployed twenty-some-things with the wealth ascribed to baby boomers who were retiring on pensions with Medicare coverage. Interestingly, the media portrayed both groups of protagonists in terms of their chronological ages. The new old rarely were portrayed as people whose passage to old age had been shaped by changes in the United States since World War II.

Finally, some of the institutions that Butler himself had launched looked vulnerable. Two decades after its founding, fretted Robert Butler, the Department of Geriatrics and Adult Development at Mount Sinai Medical Center—*the* geriatric model for training, research, and service in a U.S. medical center—was at the mercy of parochial politics and internal cutbacks. Policy decisions made in city, state, and federal governments jeopardized the department's current status and future prospects. Meanwhile, with the loss of funding from Atlantic Philanthropies amid a serious and lengthy recession that began in late 2008, Butler had to cut salaries and let go of valued employees at the International Longevity Center as he, the ILC board, and his close associates sought a new place to call home.

Butler knew full well that the intellectual, political, and organizational battles ahead of him were going to be difficult. He could have stepped aside. With some diffidence he told me of his pride in all that he had done. But Butler had worked too hard to stop fighting now; as much as he enjoyed spending time with his daughters, grandchildren, and friends, he did not see these bonds as enough to sustain him until the end of his days. Butler had spent decades trying to persuade audiences that late life (including his own) was rich in accrued insights, experiences, and potential. So he continued to proclaim that societies could ill afford to denigrate or abandon people on the basis of chronological age. Making due allowances for differences in personalities and capacities, Butler believed that most elders could adapt to changing circumstances. Through trial and error older Americans could figure out how to thrive, not merely to survive. His task was to convince people of all ages that older people demonstrably had resources beneficial to society. The Longevity Revolution had vouchsafed a win-win situation for everyone.

Butler, after all, personified the very strengths, especially human resiliency, to hammer this theme home: he had mastered the art of living and growing beyond mere survival. He had overcome loss of family and farm as a child of the Great Depression. Over his lifetime he matured as a scientist who delighted in discovering positive findings about mechanisms and processes of normal and healthy aging. Confident of the validity of scientific evidence that buttressed his presentations, he engaged in a persistent, forceful campaign to attack stereotypical images and unsubstantiated assumptions about the capacities and capabilities associated with advancing years. "I think a lot of older people are sitting on their asses, playing golf, and not making a contribution to society," he opined a few days before he died (Tapper, 2010). This is not how Butler intended to live. In late life he revealed more of his personal side in presentations and interviews, hopeful that his persona and words would sway minds.

Butler tried to improve elder care by reiterating the basics that he presented in *The Longevity Prescription*. His advice to health-care professionals was equally direct. In an age of iconic superspecialists, he stressed the value of good communication with patients. He urged caregivers to listen to older people's self-assessments. Primary-care physicians should collaborate with nurses, social workers, dentists, occupational therapists, and paraprofessionals who were committed to improving quality of life and reducing illness through preventive measures. Keenly aware that dying was part of living, Butler wanted members of interdisciplinary geriatric teams to include specialists in palliative care.

He invariably found places to affirm an upbeat answer to the question, *Why Survive?* Cognizant of various barriers to well-being in late life, he maintained the same take-away point: reaching old age afforded Americans additional chances to enjoy meaningful lives. An elder now in every sense, he was confident that he had the inner resources and network of friends and associates to plunge into endeavors that gave him satisfaction— even if circumstances were less auspicious than he had anticipated that they would be when he won the Pulitzer Prize in the prime of life. "Butler's greatest accomplishment was to help convince seniors that they could be their own most effective champions" (Laursen, 2010).

Rarely missing a chance to talk about the critical roles older people had to play, especially in the midst of population aging, Butler tirelessly granted interviews and traveled far and wide to deliver keynote addresses at professional gatherings. "Aging is a triumph, not a tragedy," he told a conference jointly sponsored by the American Society on Aging and the National Council on the Aging in March 2010. Building on his thesis in *The Longevity Revolution*, he made his case for productive aging and the New Gerontology on two fronts, economics and biology. He named the creation of Social Security and the National Institute on Aging as two notable achievements in his lifetime (Russo, 2010:1–2).

Meanwhile he eagerly embarked on new projects that (he deemed) fit his agenda. He joined Mayor Michael Bloomberg's efforts to revise the federal poverty index to take account of high housing costs in New York. (Since rents there consume roughly 45 percent of seniors' disposable income, Butler surmised that more needy elders lived in the boroughs than reported.) The project, he hoped, would generate more accurate data concerning the full extent of old-age poverty in metropolitan areas.

Butler never stopped initiating new ventures. After meeting and casually exchanging ideas with Katherine Freund during a break at a conference, he (true to form) tried to help her organization, iTNAmerica, plan ways to provide better transportation for seniors. In Butler's opinion, Freund and her colleagues were creating a new field of research on aging, which should be developed. Once he became a member of iTNAmerica's board of advisers, Butler proposed operational changes, wrote on Freund's behalf for a federal appropriation, and invited her to make a presentation at the International Longevity Center's offices to members of the World Health Organization. "He just gave," Freund declared after Butler died. "I will miss him. A very, very kind and generous man" (Freund, 2010).

Much of Butler's attention in 2009 and 2010 was consumed in ensuring the ILC's survival. He negotiated with officials to transfer the center to Columbia University's Mailman School of Public Health. There he could count on support from the dean, Dr. Linda Fried, and his long-time associate,

Dr. John Wallis Rowe. Butler also looked forward to strengthening ties with senior faculty associated with the university's international centers and its School of Social Work. Calendar entries indicate that he made time in and out of New York for reunions with family and friends. Sometimes his engagements were playful: with Dr. Aubrey de Grey, among others, Butler participated in a panel discussion of longevity research after a screening of *To Age or Not to Age*" at New York's Leonard Nimoy Thalia Theater (Snapshots, 2010).

Along the way, Butler received significant honors for his accomplishments. The University of Southern California and the University of Gothenburg in Sweden gave him honorary degrees. Butler and Myrna Lewis were inducted into the American Society on Aging Hall of Fame in 2005; he also received the Institute of Medicine's Leinhard Medal. Friends and foundations celebrated his eightieth birthday at the Metropolitan Club with a gala entitled A Great Human Achievement. Butler was particularly proud to receive the Heinz Award for the Human Condition "for advancing the rights and needs of the nation's aging citizenry and enhancing the quality of life for elderly Americans." He used his acceptance speech to recapitulate his view of the state of gerontology: "Many important adjustments, however imperfect and incomplete, have already been made," he stated. "But there is much still to be accomplished. . . . Fears of dependency, dementia, aging and death contribute to the avoidance of the topic of aging and encourage ageism, prejudice against age" ("Heinz Awards," 2003).

Besides his work at the ILC, Butler looked forward to arranging trips abroad with his grandchildren (a practice he began with Myrna) as he made plans for future travel and international speeches. So he did not mention his shoulder pain when he had dinner in late June with Dr. Barbara Paris, his friend and personal physician. Two days later, however, he presented himself at Mount Sinai. His death epitomized the "compression of morbidity" that Dr. James Fries (1983) predicted would become the norm in later years. Paris quickly determined that Butler had acute leukemia. "The ensuing transition, over the next few days, from a more than full-time work and social calendar, to end-of-life was unfathomably brief," Paris observed (2010). "That's how Bob always wanted it to be, and with love and support from his family, that's how it was. Even in his death, he left no stone unturned, leaving his brain to the Johns Hopkins Medical Institution for Alzheimer's Research." Butler's family was at his side when he died on July 4, 2010. His long-time assistant, Morriseen Barmore, noted that the stress seemed to leave his face as fireworks burst over the city.

The outpouring of tributes, reminiscences, and affection appearing on both sides of the Atlantic after Butler's death was extraordinary. "I always thought Bob Butler would live forever," Trudy Lieberman (McDavid, 2010) wrote movingly in *Columbia Journalism Review*. "After all, he was Mr. Live A Long Life, and preached the gospel of helping Americans do just that." Emma Brown (2010) concluded her lengthy obituary in the *Washington Post* with Butler's encomium to his grandmother, who "first showed him the fortitude of older people under stressful conditions." Writing in *smartplanet*, Dana Blankenhorn (2010) wrote that "you probably never heard of Robert Neil Butler . . . but if your family is like mine he transformed it." In an E-News network on generations, Paul Kleyman (2010) compared his friend to "a sequoia whose thick branches reached out to reporters even in remote reaches of journalism." Mike Magee, MD, a senior vice president of Pennsylvania Hospital in Philadelphia, reprinted previous articles on aging in his blog, *Health Commentary*, over a two-week period; Magee's "seminar on aging" was meant to honor Butler, "the unparalleled leader of geriatrics in America" (2010). Besides posting its own tribute, the International Longevity Center circulated obituaries from the *Los Angeles Times*, the *Guardian* (U.K.), and *Time* as well as remembrances composed through channels as diverse as the New York State Office for the Aging, the *Hindu*, *Mother Jones*, and *MedPage Today* (Hyland, 2010).

THE MEASURE OF A MAN

The depth of affection Butler's daughters expressed about their father is the fundamental measure of the man's capacity to love and be loved. "We love; we work, we raise our families," Sidney Poitier wrote in *The Measure of a Man*. "Those are the areas of significance in our individual lives" (2000:168). The outpouring of love was palpable in countless ways, notably at the memorial service his children arranged at All Souls Unitarian Church in September 2010. (Myrna Lewis had chosen this place for her memorial service in 2005; two years later Butler met with the senior minister to discuss his own eventual service.) Alexandra Butler sang her dad's favorite song to several hundred individuals in the congregation, many of whom had traveled from Washington, the West Coast, and abroad to pay their respects. "You were my go-to Dad," declared Cynthia Butler Gleason:

> Did you know that I attribute some of my best qualities, my stick-to-it-ive-ness, organizational skills and discipline to you, watching you operate in the world, and seeing how much it meant to others that they could count on your always. You taught me how to get a job well done, and about self-sufficiency, and the importance of maintaining relationships over time.

The family invited close associates and friends to speak, including Baroness Sally Greengross, colleagues from the ILC (Executive Director Ev Dennis, Morriseen Barmore, and Mal Schecter, who had worked with him since his NIA days); fellow geriatricians (Jack Rowe, Barbara Paris, and Diana Meier), Bob Maynard's daughter Nancy, and me. The Gerontological Society of America arranged a second memorial service at its November 2010 meeting, which featured Marie Bernard, Robert Binstock, H. R. Moody, Nora OBrien-Suric, and "Fox" Wetle.

Testimonials at these events, coupled with tributes from former medical students, foundation heads, and coworkers, attest to Butler's remarkable mentoring. He tirelessly counseled, nurtured, and supported individuals. He wanted to bring out their best so that, in due course, they would become leaders in the fields of geriatrics and gerontology. Some relationships with mentees matured into partnerships of equals—such as those with Jack Rowe, Barbara Paris, Diana Meier, Howard Fillit, and Christine Cassel. Collaborations with Rose Dobrof, Caleb Finch, Rick Moody, Jay Olshansky, and Kathleen Woodward (to mention a few) developed into friendships as well. Unlike many busy men, Butler took pride in his ability to maintain personal contacts over the phone, trips, and correspondence. Beyond this large network were individuals he never met—people who through his speeches and writings learned about productive and healthy aging or gained insights about love and sex after sixty.

Butler became a modern-day Mentor, who like the Greek god Minerva, listened seriously to young people, offered advice, and was prepared to plunge off the cliff with a mentee to reach a notable goal. Yet gifted mentoring does not fully account for Butler's success in advancing the field of aging. Mentoring, after all, tends to be a dyadic process, wherein each bond takes on a character of its own depending on the dynamics of the relationships. Butler profoundly pierced the hearts of men and women who became prominent gerontologists, geriatricians, scientists, journalists, teachers, and public servants. His real impact lay in his ability to stir the imaginations of those beyond that circle, however. Such influence goes beyond lives he directly touched.

Given all that has been written about the man since his death, it is tempting to argue that Butler almost singlehandedly altered the course of research on aging, intellectually and otherwise. The value associates and strangers ascribe to his accomplishments as a medical scientist, advocate, educator, globetrotter, and wordsmith are extraordinary. Butler's standing as a giant in gerontology and geriatrics, nonetheless, does not need meeting the criteria of Thomas Carlyle's "Great Man Theory" (1888), which postulated that heroic characters can shape historical events by dint of their charisma, wisdom, intelligence or Machiavellian designs. Carlyle's theory has long gone out of vogue. "The forces of history are far bigger than any democracy's individual voices, however loud or widely disseminated," *New York Times* critic Frank Rich reminds us (2011). Another reason to resist apotheosizing "great men" is that it tempts us to ignore or minimize the setbacks, mistakes, and character flaws that beset our genuine heroes. Like virtually any notable figure who made a difference in postwar America, Butler did not succeed in all he undertook.

It is worth reviewing Butler's life alongside biographies of contemporary luminaries. Rather than focus exclusively on people's attainments, perhaps we should pay attention to unanticipated obstacles or turns of events that can dampen lifelong accomplishments. Three comparisons suffice. To begin: JFK's assassination and the eclipse of Keynesian economics, for instance, cut short the long career of John Kenneth Galbraith (1908–2006) as a proponent of political liberalism (Parker, 2005). Then there is Sargent Shriver (1915–2011), who rightly deserves respect for his successes as the first director of the Peace Corps and the Office of Economic Opportunity as well as his work with his wife in creating the Special Olympics. Shriver's ties to the Kennedys, however, paradoxically diminished his ability to forge a political identity of his own (Stossel, 2004). Finally, think of the fate of compassionate, liberal Hubert Humphrey (1911–1978), who, like Robert Butler, rose from obscure origins; Humphrey's goal of consolidating Great Society initiatives was overshadowed by Lyndon Johnson's persona and then lost in the turmoil of the 1960s (Solberg, 1984).

Despite parallels in the lives of Butler, Galbraith, Shriver, and Humphrey, there are of course many differences. Butler was neither a Harvard economist nor a blueblood lawyer nor a politician. Other biographical comparisons, with figures in Butler's circle of friends, might prove more edifying.

Consider the career of Betty Friedan, whose *The Feminine Mystique* (1963) and *The Fountain of Age* (1993) made her one of the nation's most incisive critics of gender inequities. Friedan galvanized the women's movement. At Butler's urging, she formulated a feminist critique designed to undermine ageism. Like Butler, she based her cogent arguments for fundamental societal reforms on facts that she systematically had filed away. Unlike Butler, she had a difficult personality. Her anger inspired and provoked listeners, whereas Butler rarely voiced the rage and sarcasm sometimes evident in his writings and private conversations (Woodward, 2002).

On balance Betty Friedan's claim to being designated a public intellectual was stronger than Butler's. Consistently, using gender as her lens, she could mobilize a wide range of support and controversy. Butler knew that he was not so fortunate: "Nobody wants to talk about aging," he revealingly told a reporter in 2009 (Newton, 2010). "Age" and "longevity," despite Butler's efforts, were less effective frames than gender in shaping people's ideas about their identities. "How old are you?"—rarely a question posed for its own sake—usually was followed by a segue that moved discourse in a different direction. Hence the paradox: scientists and the public knew the importance of age—people were living longer and it was a convenient criterion for meting out bureaucratic entitlements—but age per se not only defined less about individuals than sex, race, ethnicity, or sexual orientation but (for most) also engendered more dread and revulsion than pride or affirmation. Butler tried but failed to resolve this paradox in the marketplace of ideas. As such, he resembles many public intellectuals who desired that words change people's outlooks and behaviors.

Butler's concepts of age resonated not only in scientific circles but also in cultural and political domains. He widely, articulately, and successfully communicated visions of our future aging selves across multiple constituencies. In these senses his career parallels those of idea brokers (Bauerlein, 2010; Bell, 1980; Kadushin, 1974; Small, 2002). Yet his life story differs from those of public intellectuals in postwar America. He was not an independent scholar; he did not write regularly for publications such as *Harper's*, *Commentary*, *Dissent*, or the *New York Review of Books*. At heart an optimist, Dr. Butler never presented himself (like most public intellectuals) as an alienated, marginalized critic, preoccupied with the malaise of societal decline or hopelessness about the future.

Nor was Butler associated with any readily identifiable subset of the nation's intelligentsia. He did not live the life of a detached intellectual in upstate New York like philosopher and urban critic Lewis Mumford (Hughes & Hughes, 1990). Nor did he relish being a polymath pundit and deft policy maker like Senator Daniel Patrick Moynihan (Hodgson, 2000; Schoen, 1979). He did not write pungently like Todd Gitlin (1993), a former leader of Students for Democratic Society who offered critiques of modern-day American culture.

Having spent virtually his entire career between Washington and Manhattan, Butler claimed no regional affinities such as identified Southern Agrarians, the twelve writers who bemoaned the loss of southern identity to industrialization. His relationship with professional groups such as the American Medical Association was at best cordial, since the organization rarely supported his positions on geriatrics and health-care financing. His interests and politics differed ideologically and temperamentally from those of New York Jews who began to reposition themselves from socialism to neoconservatism in the late 1960s. While he harbored political ambitions and held strong views about racial inequality, injustice, foreign policy, and national politics, Butler hewed to age-related issues in writings and speeches. Nor did he embellish a distinctive mode of discourse as did African American intellectuals as different in outlook as Cornel West (Boynton, 1991), Peter Gomes ("Remember," 2011), and Henry Louis Gates ("Henry," 2011) when they addressed broad social, economic, and political themes.

If it is too much to claim that he was a public intellectual, a case can be made that Butler rightly earned respect and credibility in the public sphere because of his scientific credentials. Articulate scientists and physicians generally command respect in the media and enjoy influence among idea brokers. Butler's solid command of theories and themes of aging calls to mind the breadth with which psychologist G. Stanley Hall (Lepore, 2011), Albert Einstein, Stephen Hawking, Lewis Thomas (Weissmann, 2010), or C. Everett Koop enthralled audiences (Jacoby, 1987; Michael, 2000). To the extent that people were interested in learning more about how humans grow older, they could count on Butler punctuating erudition with memorable, upbeat phrases.

By the time Robert Butler gained fame for *Why Survive?* (1975), however, the golden era for public intellectuals was waning. Few nowadays can meet Richard Posner's definition that "a public intellectual expresses himself in a way that is accessible to the public, and the focus of his expression is on matters of general public concern of (or inflected by) a political or ideological cast" (2001:35). The best-known figures today, critics bemoan, tend to be publicity-driven pseudo-intellectuals or "talking heads." Their penchant for risk taking, for challenging conventional wisdom over national values and public norms, it seems, has declined in inverse proportion to securing tenured positions. "Where are the independent intellectuals now?" wondered Michael Ignatieff (1997), the liberal who himself migrated from international academic pinnacles with mixed results into the grit of Canadian provincial politics: "The death of the intellectual has left a void in the centre of public life. In place of thought, we have opinion; in place of argument, we have journalism; in place of polemic we have personality profiles; in place of reputation, we have celebrity" (see also Bramwell, 2010; Giroux, 2011). Within the changing milieu of how and where ideas matter, Robert Butler emerges as a visionary, not a public intellectual.

"Bob's purpose was to be a visionary leader, to inspire others to believe in better care for older people and take up the charge," observed Nora OBrien-Suric (2010) in the John A. Hartford Foundation blog. "It took a leader to prepare the way; it takes an entire workforce to build a better society for older people. . . . Let's honor Bob by working together towards our common goal." OBrien-Suric's invitation to collective action presupposes resolution of a fundamental question: did Butler truly succeed in developing a big-picture vision of age and aging that will mobilize large numbers of gerontologists and citizens in the years ahead?

To mount big pictures requires visionaries to choose durable frames. "Frames influence the ways in which we think about things, emphasizing some aspects of a phenomenon and deemphasizing others" (Cappella & Jamieson, 1997; Lambino, 2009). Contemporary communications experts, political scientists, politicians, pollsters, and marketers know the importance of framing. Walter Lippmann observed in *Public Opinion* that "the way the world is imagined determines at any particular moment what men will do" (1922:25). Frames, which rely on apt metaphors as filters and constructing perceptions that play to people's emotions and principles, serve to organize a hierarchy of principles that ideally persist over time (Fairhurst, 2006; FrameWorks Institute, 2002; Lakoff, 2004).

At least three changes in postwar American culture complicate the task of framing any policy issue or big idea, frustrating even skilled communicators like Butler. First, high-brow and low-brow commentators agree that popular discourse, particularly ideas and words shaping political debates, has been dumbed down in the United States (Benen, 2011; Fornal, 2011; Rockefeller, 2011). Forrest Gump had it right: "Stupid is as stupid does" (Burnett, 2009). Present-day critics probably give too much credit to the influence of the Tea Party and the widespread use of broken words on cellular devices for the sorry state of current affairs. Historians have traced a dogged tradition of anti-intellectualism in U.S. history dating back to the Jacksonian era, if not before (Hofstadter, 1963; Lim, 2008).

Second, there was enthusiasm on college campuses and university research centers for developing cross-cutting fields of inquiry during the 1950s and 1960s, though departments even then claimed most deans' attention and budget. Now, interdisciplinary programs like gerontology by and large languish. Disciplines in the sciences and foreign languages have subdivided (and some, like geography, have imploded) as leaders in academic settings put a premium on specialization whose worth is measured by articles' impact in top-flight journals and the size of grants supporting research. Greater numbers of undergraduates pursue business majors than liberal-arts degrees. This fragmentary pattern is evident among experts and laypersons who rely on metrics to assess knowledge making instead of debating ideas.

Third, the postwar me-too generation discounts the value of past traditions and denies the importance of future contingencies to the present. "We are fast losing the sense of historical continuity, the sense of belonging to a succession of generations originating in the past and stretching into the future," Christopher Lasch pointed out in *The Culture of Narcissism*. "The waning of the sense of historical time—in particular, the erosion of any strong concern for posterity" perturbed Lasch (1979:5). To the extent that people entertain the prospects of "future shock," they focus mainly on imminent crises that demand immediate attention. Attending to slow-moving doomsday scenarios—such as the possible dire consequences of population aging—is put off until they reach catastrophic proportions.

The issue of old-age entitlements is a case in point. In the 1980s, when it appeared that Social Security would run out of money unless lawmakers quickly shored up its financing, a bipartisan group of legislators and policy makers saved the day with a package of benefit reductions, tax increases, and bureaucratic legerdemain (Laursen, 2012). Some felt that more radical steps had to be taken, given the graying of America in general and the aging of the baby boom cohort in particular. Peter Peterson for the next three decades attacked Social Security, Medicare, and Medicaid as "outdated and bloated programs" (2010, 1999). As a former secretary of commerce, chairman of Lehman Brothers, and president of the Concord Coalition,

Peterson had the financial resources and media access to disseminate his views.

Butler thought that his friend Peter Peterson went too far in blaming recent global trends in population aging for an unsustainable world economy likely to erupt in generational warfare. Butler agreed, however, that it was prudent for Americans to take steps that might mitigate the negative impact of seemingly inexorable demographic trends. He shared Peterson's concern that America's reluctance to make long-term investments in infrastructure would broaden an "innovation gap" between the U.S. and emerging economies (Fallows, 2011; Redlener, 2009; Schwartz, 2011; Vella, 2008). Yet Butler considered this challenge to be less urgent than empowering men and women of all ages (and especially elders) to engage in productive aging.

That Butler agreed at points with Peterson complicated his framing of an argument. (The same might be said of his sparring with Aubrey de Gray, whom he also liked, though he did not think much of his ideas.) Butler sought to be a consensus builder at a time in which the media preferred to air controversy. He often set forth nuanced arguments because he refused to offer only sound bites. He tried mightily to focus on priorities as he underscored salient age-related changes in his narrative. Even when he recognized that his message was not getting across, he held his ground as he struggled to increase awareness of late-life potentials.

Darkly describing the United States to me as a "nation of small thought," Butler often had to express ideas about age and aging to audiences indifferent, often resistant, to his message. He understood the difference between delivering a sound bite and constructing a narrative.

Butler was a master at translating pithy ideas into plain English. His descriptions of "healthy aging" and "productive aging" surely were plain enough even in a marketplace of ideas where dumbed-down language prevailed. So too was "ageism," which deliberately played off "racism" and "sexism." The analogy, he knew, did not quite work: skin color and genitalia rarely undergo changes, but everyone who lives long enough becomes old. Other terms that he coined may yet become popular. "Shortgevity," the loss of life expectancy in nations due to epidemics and market catastrophe, was Butler's clever twist on "longevity" (2008:362–63).

Butler neither aspired nor pretended to be a theorist. To the best of my knowledge, he never espoused a meta theory of knowledge. And while his enduring love for Columbia's Core Curriculum predisposed him to engage in interdisciplinary discussions, at heart he was a pragmatic scientist, someone interested in verifying phenomena. He preferred using his findings to develop interventions rather than philosophizing. Problem focused, Butler was results oriented. "I question how truly effective academe is in creating multi- and especially interdisciplinary programs," he noted in *The Longevity Revolution*, "yet these are just the programs we must plan and execute to solve Alzheimer's disease" (2008:142). Against the odds, he wished to work within existing structures to advance his causes.

When Butler talked about the "future," he put a human face on the construct. This is why he referred so often to baby boomers, whose numbers after World War II had forced changes in the educational system and in the marketplace. Their present and proximate prospects were unclear, however. Butler did not know whether some boomers in late life would alter postmodernism as they had transformed the 1960s, but a miserable old age awaited them, he feared, if they did not adapt. Butler hoped that boomers would be a catalyst for constructive change.

However earnestly and adeptly Butler framed images of aging, he faced many of the same issues that prevented other experts from being successful advocates for their social causes. Journalists from major TV and radio stations and the nation's leading dailies sought Butler's comments on news about aging. But these outlets no longer had a tight grip on elite audiences and revenues. The proliferation of cable networks and Internet sites hungry to grow market segments required news sources for hot-button topics. In this new milieu Butler's reputation as one of the world's leading gerontologists no longer accorded him deference or prime-time access. He had to compete for space in the public square with many other people who were eager to share their views and prejudices about growing older. Everyone, it seemed, was entitled to share her or his opinions in blogs and on local talk shows. Because the ideological bite of some pundits was more sensational than Butler's moderate tone, unknowns sometimes replaced him in front of cameras and media broadcasts.

These realities, wherein the media's immediate demands for newsworthiness took precedence over experts' needs for accuracy and caution, complicated choices that Butler and other gerontologists faced. How should he select features of age and aging that would enable people to grasp what he considered to be essential in apprehending the dynamics of growing older? Fundamentally, from the start of his career, he offered an optimistic message about gerontology and longevity. Yet he knew that the promise of scientific research on aging would not and could not be fully realized for some time. This left him with a twofold challenge.

First, since the beginning of recorded history, commentators had expressed a wide range of antithetical notions about the meanings and experiences of growing older. Positive and negative images have clashed across centuries: for every Ciceronian paean about wise heads was a disparaging ode by Juvenal. Alarmist rhetoric flamed audiences' fears and anxieties about growing older. Scenarios that sounded too rosy invited skepticism that dissolved into despair. And yet presentations of old age as a variegated stage tended to burden audiences with imagining future scenarios by turns ambivalent, nonlinear, or paradoxical (Achenbaum & Albert, 1995; Booth, 1992; Cole & Winkler, 1994).

Second, research on aging did not emerge as a bona fide field of inquiry until after World War II. Some scientists still question gerontology's legitimacy as an area of study, as well as the value of geriatrics as a distinctive domain of the health sciences. Many wish to subsume gerontology under other branches of knowledge and delegate elder care to internists, neurologists, and family physicians. Even when the science of longevity is accorded a niche, it rarely attracts the attention enjoyed by cognitive behavioral science or the biology of sex. Young people typically define aging in terms of their grandparents. No wonder classes on aging suffer in comparison to computer science, women's studies, or neuroscience.

Worse, there is a nagging sense that gerontology is at best a pseudoscience. Many of the domain's forbears, after all, were charlatans, alchemists, and hucksters. The origins of the present-day anti-aging industry lie in lotions, contraptions, and pills sold in Conestoga wagons. Eminent scientists occasionally contributed to gerontology's dubious reputation: Elie Metchnikoff, the Nobel laureate who coined the term "gerontology," for instance, recommended daily consumption of yogurt to extend life. Metchnikoff's intriguing remedy simply does not work (Post & Binstock, 2004). Other panaceas—such as large doses of x-rays, glandular implants, or over-the-counter nostrums, including many remedies touted as anti-aging medicine—have not lived up to expectations. Ageism triumphs in this milieu: nihilist critiques seem justifiable whenever science fails to deliver anticipated remedies.

However Butler framed his argument, his message was bound to clash with others' misstatements and biases, past and present. To be persuasive, he had to ground his vision in the best scientific knowledge at his disposal. Despite Butler's attractive persona, his thoughts on old age and longevity did not dispel the notion, widely held, that "geriatrics is in part responsible, albeit involuntarily and with the best of intentions, for covering up the afflictions of old age" (Bobbio, 2001:23–24).

Commentators often dichotomize old age in order to underline the shift from healthful maturity to dependency with advancing years. "There are two diverging narratives about old age that are competing to replace the 'golden years' vision of retirement as perpetual R&R," claimed columnist Ellen Goodman (2011). This has always been a strategy historically. Artists and writers in ancient Greece distinguished between a "green old age" and "senectitude or second childhood." Others juxtaposed Ganymede (the eternal youth) and Tithonos (the soldier whose extraordinary longevity ended in decrepitude). Butler's dear friend gerontologist Bernice Neugarten (1974) contrasted the "young old" with the "old old."

Sometimes experts choose to accentuate the young olds' positive attributes as a counterpoint to negative images of aging. Thus Peter Laslett (1989), creating an analogy to Neugarten's schema, focused on the vitality and potentials of men and women in the so-called Third Age. Butler, unlike Laslett or the Eriksons, chose not to invoke stage models. He questioned concepts of the life course that posited that individuals passed through one set of challenges to the next in a lock-step manner. This is why early on he rejected the Eriksons' paradigm, which set forth a sequence of distinctive stages psychological in nature.

Stages bracketed by ages, Butler felt, were dubious, given the varieties of circumstances with advancing years. Chronology per se could not accurately predict people's mental capacities, health statuses, or social conditions. Instead Butler believed that old age was neither an extension of middle age nor the last, abysmal transition to death. To his mind, the future consequences of the Longevity Revolution should inspire gratitude, not despair. "Life has to be based on hope and expectation of a positive future," he told Ronni Bennett in 2008. "When that future is removed as in the case of old age it builds dissatisfaction, disappointment, and depression. This obviously affects our culture."

Butler readily conceded to Bennett that "we are a long way from having conquered the prejudices regarding aging." With a positive spin he described age-related deficits. He shared the optimism of historian-physician Gerald Gruman, who declared that "the aging population does have a future, as it becomes reengaged at the frontier of modern cultural adaptation and realization through historical time" (1978:380). The best available scientific evidence concerning physical conditions in late life, moreover, seemed to justify Butler's position. "Older Americans are generally healthy," declared John Rowe and Robert Kahn in their MacArthur study, *Successful Aging* (1998:18; see also Sarkistan, 2002). "Even in advanced old age, an overwhelming majority of the elderly population have little functional disability, and the proportion that is disabled is being whittled away over time" (Rowe & Kahn, 1998).

Gerontologists in Europe, meanwhile, were urging colleagues to focus research on the Fourth Age, wherein people with radically diminished physical or mental competencies lose their autonomy and must rely on others for basic needs. As a consequence of the Longevity Revolution, they claimed, more and more people were living long enough to endure diminutions in cognition, mobility, and resiliency. "The Fourth Age commences when half the original 'birth cohort' is no longer alive," declared Paul B. Baltes, director of the Max Planck Institute for Human Development in Berlin. "The Fourth Age makes explicit the biological shortcomings of the human organism—and based on current evidence there is little hope of the oldest ages becoming the veritable 'golden age'" (Baltes, 2003; see also Baltes & Smith, 2003; Baltes & Mayer, 2001; Gilleard & Higgs, 2010, 2011; Johnson, 2011). To them the Longevity Revolution did not create an additional *stage* of life so much as broaden *states* of incapacity.

Butler, aware of work by Baltes and others, hedged bets about "our future selves": "I am always a guarded optimist and I do think the baby boomers, a very large generation, may be transformative. I am not sure they will be able to benefit as much themselves but that they will contribute to improved quality of life for the generations that follow" (Bennett, 2011). In retrospect, Butler's qualification did not stretch enough to embrace the Fourth Age. A rising cohort of American critics presented an alternative portrait of age to his guarded optimism concerning the power of science to ensure health and meaning in the extra years of life resulting from the Longevity Revolution. Butler's references to frailty in his papers with Dr. Fillit are no match for the vividly depressing images that Simone de Beauvoir in *The Coming of Age* (1971) or Susan Jacoby in *Never Say Die* (2011) presented. These commentators characterized aging as synonymous with decline, which fans a fear surfacing in middle age that persists over time. Butler was correct in not delineating stages of aging. Still, he should have asserted fully that in the Fourth Age states of incapacity multiplied at advanced ages.

Old age remains terra incognita, an elongated period of time by turns cherished, endured, and feared. In his last years Butler knew he still had much to write and do to sustain his ebullient view that aging bestowed gifts beyond mere survival. Fully aware that ageism and various dementias prevented millions from benefiting from the Longevity Revolution, he never gave up hope that science's triumph over the diseases and debilities of later years ultimately would disarm the doomsday prophets of age.

At his death Butler left the rest of us an unfulfilled strategy for advancing the new gerontology to serve the common good. Should we baby boomers pursue his age prescription? Should we fight ageism by integrating research, training, and advocacy? Should we be bolder than Butler in accentuating the benefits of late life in the Longevity Revolution, by elaborating on the fullness of love that can ripen in old age or the richness of experiences to be shared with peers and young people? Or must we for our own sakes rough up his argument, highlighting various vicissitudes of age that reduce people who live too long to mere survival or worse?

※ ※ ※ ※ ※

Butler leaves behind an extraordinary set of achievements that do not neatly translate into an unequivocal call to arms. It remains for us, the baby boomers and those who follow, to look forward with eyes on the past and the present. We invariably will build on Butler's legacy, but we may have to redirect the course of action to achieve his goals.

Accordingly, it makes sense to compare Butler's life and accomplishments to those of W. E. B. DuBois (1869–1963), the African American trailblazer who sought to improve conditions and opportunities for another marginalized segment of the population (Lewis, 2001). In opposition to Booker T. Washington, who thought that black people had to accommodate white society, DuBois wrote landmark books (such as *The Souls of Black Folk*) and created institutions (such as the NAACP) to advance equal rights for African Americans. Like Butler, DuBois was an energetic pragmatist who incorporated the best available scientific methods into research. While focusing on matters of race, he also supported women's rights and the peace movement and, in his Pan-Africanism, embraced global issues. There are differences: unlike Butler, DuBois embraced unpopular political positions; he was a socialist who blamed capitalism for racism.

One other parallel cinches the comparison between DuBois and Butler. DuBois died before the passage of the Civil Rights Act. Martin Luther King, Jr., not DuBois, framed a narrative of justice that moved a nation. So, too, Butler's vision of aging America will find its full measure in words and deeds chosen by boomers and our successors to galvanize public awareness and appreciation for the significance of age in every facet of life.

EPILOGUE

"Now we have both past work as a foundation and new scientific tools offering hope that we may soon have a more prolonged, vigorous, and productive life and added longevity," Butler predicted in *The Longevity Revolution* (2008:187). "During the twenty-first century, the century of the life sciences, longevity science should truly come of age." Determining the best approaches to harvest the fruits of Butler's productivity becomes ongoing legacy work for current and future students of human aging.

Our task is to build on Butler's capacious and optimistic vision of aging, in which young and old would grow into healthful, productive elderhood, clothed in all its special mysteries, exigencies, ambiguities, and contingencies. Achieving this objective, Butler knew, entailed more than repackaging late life's meanings and experiences. The Longevity Revolution demands concerted political action: as we uproot prejudices about growing older, we must invest in research on aging and develop policies to empower all age-groups to prepare for their future selves. The New Gerontology encourages post–World War II cohorts to be stewards of an intergenerational compact, which has been undervalued and threatened in recent decades amid pressures to cut basic health and social services. Butler invites us to imagine and actualize how diverse facets of aging present fresh, productive ways to fulfill our civic duties and moral responsibilities to one another, at home and abroad.

Butler highlighted incentives for us to act in our best interest. If we succeed in harnessing the Longevity Revolution, we can ensure that men and women of all ages have access to health-care professionals who promote healthful living. We can broaden (adult) educational opportunities to support careers and enrich lives. We can reorder institutional priorities to conserve and sustain livable environments in our local communities and globally.

Robert Butler has passed the baton. We are called to modify and embellish ideas and practices that he advanced. His gerontological imagination, themes, and modus operandi offer prescriptions for healthfulness, psychological and interpersonal growth, and productivity. Butler constructed a paradigm for a New Gerontology that links biomedical discoveries to intellectual, political, economic, and social issues related to old age and aging.

Building on his themes, I propose to reframe Butler's vision of aging through a threefold agenda that can advance his legacy: (1) to incorporate life-course perspectives into gerontological theory building, (2) to tap elders' energy and wisdom amid a global environmental crisis, and (3) to extirpate ageism. Addressing these issues has intellectual, practical, and beneficial consequences for boomers and younger persons who are growing older.

1. *Studies of old age and aging require life-course perspectives.* Dr. Butler sometimes expressed regret that he did not situate ideas about healthy, productive aging often enough in a life-course context. This perspective, in my opinion, too rarely informed the theoretical moorings of his biomedical or behavioral projects. He nonetheless recognized the construct's relevance to gerontology. "A life course perspective seeks to prevent during infancy, childhood, and youth the diseases of old age," he observed in *The Longevity Revolution* (2008:228). "It can foster an appreciation of the dynamic processes of aging, which counters a stereotypic and negative image." Butler grasped the significance of life-course perspectives on aging research in papers by historian Tamara K. Hareven (1994) and sociologist Glen Elder (1999), whose work he funded at NIA.

He and Myrna Lewis (1986:ix) realized, ten years after writing *Sex After Sixty*, that "worries about bodily changes with age, fears about impotence and loss of sexual attractiveness, anxieties about social acceptance in a culture that idealizes youth, relationship problems over time, and other issues—were as much a concern for the middle aged as for those who were older." Rather than enlarge their best seller, the couple wrote a new book, *Midlife Love Life*, which went through several editions.

At least two other approaches to life-course perspectives on aging are available. First, Alexandra Close launched the New California (now America) Media in 1996 to unite people of different ethnicities, youth, elders, and other marginalized groups through media outlets that influence policy makers (Kleyman, 2010). Second, in keeping with Butler's concept of Life Review, collective biographies have been written about selected groups of artists (Galenson, 2006; Sohm, 2007) and members of scientific communities (Brumfield, 2008; Normile, 2004).

To my mind, gerontologists must assess continuities and changes that occur early in life while probing the dynamics of aging. Turf battles with pediatricians, adolescent psychologists, and marriage counselors undoubtedly will ensue. The price is worth it. After all, gerontologists who deploy continuity theories of aging already analyze developments in childhood and youth and address critical links between middle age and old age (Atchley, 1983; Maddox, 1968). As we refine scientifically valid, age-based criteria for assessing late maturity, some will continue to seek hitherto elusive bio-markers or genetic tests (Grant, 2011; Willard & Ginsberg, 2009). Others will stress the importance of rituals and rites of passage (Sankar, 2011). Still others will explicate differences by race and gender in relation to age and disability (Campbell, 1993; Hatch, 2000; Moen, Dempster-McClain, & Williams, 1992; Pifer & Bronte, 1986).

Above all, students of late-life development must think out of the box, integrating life-course perspectives into studies of individual and societal aging. The thirty additional years of life that Americans on average have gained over the past century are spread across the life course. This longevity bonus makes obsolete the traditional three boxes of life—school, work, and retirement. Extra years realign virtually every institutional arrangement

(Achenbaum, 2012; Carstensen, 2009; Rowe, forthcoming). Accommodations have already been made for me and other baby boomers. Teachers and taxpayers had to build new schools as we passed through educational systems. Women in my cohort gave difference valance to jobs and families in career decisions. Boomers pursued spiritual paths and volunteering opportunities unimaginable to our grandparents. We shortly will renegotiate end-of-life decisions with families and health-care providers.

Besides paying greater attention to events from infancy through middle age, U.S. gerontologists must collaborate with geriatricians and other health-care professionals in reviewing the causes and courses of diseases and disabilities that diminish late-life capacities. Having made Alzheimer's disease a top priority at the National Institute on Aging, Butler lived long enough to witness the dramatic evolution of the scientific underpinnings of that scourge and of other dementias. New scientific evidence changed his views after he left NIA. "Aging is a risk factor, and Alzheimer's disease is a disorder of longevity," he flatly declared in *The Longevity Revolution*. "Alzheimer's, Parkinson's disease, and amyotrophic lateral sclerosis (Lou Gehrig's disease) are all diseases of longevity and result from the death of a specific set of nerve cells. In fact, these diseases may be related" (2008:127, 132). Butler's views of these related diseases came closer to those of critics (O'Connor, Prusiner, & Dychtwald, 2010).

Paradoxically, I fear that our preoccupation with Alzheimer's lulls us to ignore other mental disorders. Gerontologists should integrate life-course perspectives in updating Butler and Lewis's *Aging and Mental Health*. Depression soon will be the second highest cause of disease burden; its cost in the United States in 2003 exceeded $83 billion (Gutierrez-Lobos, 2002; Rait, 2009). Youth, women, unmarried persons, and the unemployed are most susceptible to the disease. Estimates of depression in old age range from 9 percent to 18 percent (because of sampling difficulties); the malady afflicts nearly a third of those in nursing homes. Depression contributes to suicide rates that are highest among those over age 75. The onset of depression in later years, rarely sudden, presents preclinical symptoms before physicians diagnose the disease (Berger et al., 1998; Luijendijk et al., 2008; Stek et al., 2006). Loneliness, receding social networks, chronic pain, impaired capacities (including a decreased ability to metabolize alcohol), harmful medical interactions (older people use three times the number of prescriptions as the general population), liver disease, insomnia, and anxiety disorders all contribute to substance abuse among older people. Heavy drinking is a risk factor for depression among men, which contributes to hip fractures and rates of hospital admission equal to those for myocardial infarction (Bartels et al., 2005; Merrick et al., 2008; Patterson & Jeste, 1999; Saunders et al., 1991).

We have paid too little attention to the mental status of older people, despite its palpable significance. "Medical and psychotherapeutic professions, which come most closely in contact with older people, still have not made an active commitment to their special concerns and problems," wrote Butler and Lewis in *Aging and Mental Health* (1982:17, 150). Despite efforts by the National Institute on Aging and the National Institute of Mental Health, most health-care professionals still fail decades later to provide sufficient attention to older people's mental conditions. "Mental illness (depression, alcohol dependence, and schizophrenia) are hidden diseases and impose a major burden," Butler reported in *The Longevity Revolution* (2008:345). "While psychiatric conditions are responsible for little more than 1% of deaths, they account for almost 11 percent of the disease burden worldwide." Signs of mental illness go unattended, and treatment plans usually are inadequate in later years: patient reluctance to discuss their moods parallels health-care professionals' indifference to ask. We need life-course perspectives to comprehend the prevalence of mental illness so that we can gauge and remedy its deleterious impact on quality of life with advancing age.

2. *Healthy, productive aging is gray and green.* Geriatricians and gerontologists resemble members of other academic and professional tribes; they prefer to work in isolated arenas. Unlike Butler, who over the course of his career expanded his expertise as a gero-psychiatrist and old-age advocate to a host of social issues, most researchers on aging rarely participate in conversations about such global challenges as human rights, meaningful employment, and health disparities. Doing so might validate Butler's hypothesis that increased average life expectancies generate economic

growth and wealth in aging societies. Such an emphasis could underscore the importance of age and longevity in framing issues that initially might seem removed from matters of individual and societal aging. It should bolster Butler's case for putting a human face of aging on how environmental destruction diminishes quality of life:

> The environmental movement has been extraordinarily important in bringing attention to the degradation of the environment and the need to maintain a livable biosphere. However, certain assumptions require fresh examination. . . . There is the mistaken idea that a human being is somehow artificial, or at war with that which is natural. It must be stressed that we are part of nature and have altered nature as no other animal form has ever done. We need to build a constructive alliance between nature and economic development, ensuring mutual adaptability. (2008:374)

Butler's premise that senior citizens have a stake in conserving our fragile Earth rests on self-interested idealism. "As our population ages and faces the chronic diseases of our time, [we must] think about our obligations to future generations and the quality of the world we will leave to them" (see also Schletter & Valenti, 2010). "Older people everywhere should aspire," like Butler, "to be gray and green." "Aspire" may be too tepid; we must take immediate action.

Sustaining a healthy environment promotes healthful aging. Research shows that heat waves, hurricanes, and pollutants cause older persons to suffer physiological and psychological susceptibility and social vulnerability (Gostin, 2010; Sykes & Pillemer, 2009, 2010). Environmental issues receive broader attention than age concerns, yet they too summon less remedial action than conditions warrant. Americans are not yet persuaded that the frequency of droughts, famines, and erratic temperatures points to an environmental time bomb, worsening ecological degradation. The crisis, therefore, gives aging baby boomers an opportunity to do worthwhile legacy work in gerontology while leaving something tangible and meaningful for those to come (Freedman, 2006–07; Moody & Achenbaum, forthcoming).

Summoning eco-elders to civic engagement should appeal to members of my cohort who reminisce or complete life reviews. Boomers remember the rivers, fields, and beaches of our youth. Many of us joined the Civil Rights movement and protested the war in Vietnam. Earth Day celebrations in the 1970s were part of this same civic engagement, our commitment to participate in ensuring the protection of core values. Accordingly, joining the present-day ecological movement may counterbalance stereotypes of us being "greedy geezers," graying rogues with seemingly little concern for rising generations. Confronting negative images of age and aging, in turn, requires us to redouble Butler's assault on ageism.

3. *Ageism is really gerontophobia.* Toward the end of his life, Butler repeatedly claimed that the origins of ageism were "not only rooted in historic and economic circumstances [but] they also derive from deeply held human concerns and fears about the vulnerability inherent in the later years of life." At the International Longevity Center Butler (2009:211) wanted "to document the extent to which [ageism] exists in America and elsewhere to examine the status of legislation and case law at work to overcome this prejudice. We regard our effort to transform the culture and the experience of aging as quintessential and urgent. *Ultimately, such initiatives will benefit all who would grow old.*" This is why Butler proposed a Declaration of Human Rights of Older Persons at the 2002 U.N. World Assembly on Aging.

Butler had come a long way since coining "ageism" during a *Washington Post* interview with Carl Bernstein in 1968 amid a fight over senior housing in the Capitol. Then, he drew parallels between racial and sexual prejudice and discrimination against the old. Forty years later, he understood much better how policy got enacted, how the media shaped issues, and how ideas (while invaluable) did not invariably change people's views and social conventions. Fears and prejudices of aging, he recognized, would only abate by reconstructing old age. Butler in candid moments wondered, as we talked about his life, whether he himself, now over seventy-five, had become a target of age discrimination. Ageism, he knew from empirical evidence and personal experience, can strike anyone, anytime, anywhere.

Ageism itself festers in a historical milieu much changed since the late 1960s. Racial and gender-based inequalities remain, but most Americans think twice before making racist and sexist slurs. Legislation has not eliminated discrimination against those with disabilities or suppressed homophobia, but U.S. citizens evince more tolerance than before. Intermarriage has muted religious bigotry. Yet ageism remains prominent among the last havens for expressing socially acceptable bigotry.

I think it noteworthy that Butler in late life characterized ageism as "gross and subtle, and omnipresent." In *The Longevity Revolution* he called the animus against age a "psychosocial disease" (2008:53). More than a prejudice or even a fear, as Butler once had claimed, ageism in his opinion mushroomed into a pathological illness.

In a special issue of *Generations* (2005c:84–86), Butler offered a "brief history of my encounters with this self-destructive prejudice." His article, "Ageism: Looking Back Over My Shoulder," noted his "being different from other boys by virtue of having older 'parents' who, in fact, were my grandparents." He then recounted how encounters with age prejudice in medical school and as an intern led him to do research on aging at the National Institute of Mental Health. Next he illustrated ageism in various aspects of his career, whether confronting age discrimination in the airline industry or debunking the notion of sexlessness in writing *Love and Sex After Sixty* with Myrna Lewis. "Over the years, my conception of ageism has continued to evolve," he observed. "More focus should be placed on . . . especially the second wave of baby boomers, as well as generations X and Y, to help them understand ageism and its untoward consequences."

At the end of his life, Butler expressed urgency, frustration, and anger over ageism:

> It is time to alter our deep-seated cultural sensibility and work to overcome our fear, our shunned responsibility, and harmful avoidance and denial of age. Strict legislation, as well as legal and police action against age discrimination and abuse, are essential but insufficient. We must help people deal with their fears of aging, dependency, and death, and develop a sense of the life course as a whole. (2008:58)

Those who choose to build on Butler's legacy must delve deeply into the relationship between ageism and gerontophobia. Do we dread aging more—or perhaps differently—than we express a fear of snakes, dogs, dentists, flying, chaos, frailty, or death? Do fears change with the passage of time? Why do boomers, all of whom have experienced some loss and disappointment, find it so scary to confront discomfiting situations (Bytheway, 2005; Gower, 2005; Isbell, 2009; Macnicol, 2006; Nelson, 2002)?

Butler thought that education is key in winning the battle against ageism. So do I. It is never too early to introduce "aging" into curricula. And if we can teach members of the sandwich generation to stop smoking and to set money aside for later years, why can we not prepare them for future possibilities, including the prospect that they may be marginalized by ageism? We need positive images of maturity in the media—not just portraits of extraordinarily talented and energetic characters, but those of women and men who manage to cope with adversity while making a difference in the lives of others.

In the closing paragraphs of *Why Survive?* Butler offered an action plan that remains useful as we contemplate our future selves:

> None of us know whether we have already had the best years of our lives or whether the best are yet to come. But the greatest of human possibilities remain to the very end of life—the possibilities for love and feeling, reconciliation and resolution. . . . The tragedy of old age in America is that we have made absurdity all but inevitable. We have cheated ourselves. But we still have the possibility of making life a work of art. (1975:421–22)

Life is brief and death inevitable, yet hope can pervade what remains. Growing older does not have to be meaningless or absurd. Butler believed that humans did not have to cheat or to be incredibly lucky to muster the courage and resilience to gamble on living.

This is why we must affirm the benefits that inhere in Butler's formulation of the Life Review as we follow his prescription for aging in the Longevity Revolution. Gerontologists and geriatricians are rightly concerned about probabilities in large populations. As an individual, however, I am fundamentally interested in where my life may be heading. I recognize that I must die someday, somehow, but much will occur between now and then. What terrifies me is uncertainty: I want to know how likely decline and dependence are in the offing. Having dealt with risks and uncertainty earlier in life did not brace me for what may follow. It was only when I entered the country of the old that I experienced the joys and freedom of growing older that accompany its deficits. No book, no mentor sufficiently prepared me for the very end of life.

The antidote to ageism is to take to heart Butler's observation that "the greatest of human possibilities remain to the very end of life." He knew this. He loved well all his life; his capacity for intimacy and generativity did not diminish. He recognized that love takes different forms, comes in different patterns. At the same time, he was astute and wise enough to generate new insights into forgiveness, optimism and grace. His own life is a testimony to triumphing over setbacks, being diligent and productive. Robert Butler epitomized the healthy, healthful aging he wished for others.

So it falls to boomers, whom Butler considered the litmus test of his words and deeds, to demonstrate the resilience and maturity he so admired. Now that we are in the third quarter of life, many of us find our assets as diminished as our stamina. It is foolish to pretend that some of our worst fears about aging (pain, isolation, helplessness) do not exist. At the same time we have ripened enough to be freer than ever before to ignore people's expectations and societal conventions that might dictate our choices. Somehow many of us discover that we can live as we wish, to savor intimacy and rejoice in grandchildren. We have come to understand why forgiveness trumps retaliation. We can imagine a distant future, when we are gone, in which the world could be fortified by gifts of ours that sustain and enrich others. As it was with Butler, it is "the greatest of human possibilities [that] remain" that animate us. Like him we celebrate and cultivate dreams and hopes that may come to fruition with extra years. And if so, it will be that vitality, oft underappreciated until one is old, that makes meaning possible.

appendix
PROLOGUE OR INTRODUCTION TO LIFE REVIEW

BY ROBERT N. BUTLER, 2010

Mem'ry's pointing wand, that calls the past to our exact review.
—WILLIAM COWPER, *TASK* (1784)

The author and university teacher, Patricia Hampl, wrote in 1999, "The memoir has become the signature genre of our age." There is a huge appetite for personal memoirs. But it was different in the 1950's when I arrived at the National Institute of Mental Health as a young medical scientist. At that time, the tendency to reminisce by older people was seen as a likely precursor of senile psychosis, which today we call Alzheimer's disease. The reminiscences of the old were seen as aimless wandering of mind and purposeless nostalgia likely to bore listeners, accompanied by garrulity. This negative view of reminiscence and of older persons in general was reflected in the textbooks of psychiatry and psychology of the time.

Our in-depth study of some *fifty healthy, community-resident men*, whose average age was initially 71, was carried out over an eleven-year period. Previous work had been largely conducted in chronic hospital and nursing home populations.

Our work, along with a similar study at Duke University led by Ewald "Bud" Busse, resulted in major clarifications of the nature of healthy aging. *This body of work, for example, found that much attributed to aging is in fact a function of disease, social adversity, economic status and even per-sonality.* This revision of serious misinterpretations demonstrated that healthy, community resident older persons could be in good mental and physical health. It staked a claim for the possibilities of positive, effective aging, later called, variously, productive, successful, vital, active, healthy, positive and optimal aging. Our work helped eliminate many stereotypes such as the idea that the older people are hypochondriacal and that senility is an inevitable consequence of growing older.

The NIMH studies of human aging also suggested new ways of thinking about memory in the later years. As I listened to these wonderful healthy volunteers, *I came to realize that when they were reminiscing, it was not due to brain pathology at all but reflected an important effort to come to terms with the lives they had led. I postulated that there is a natural, per-haps universal, phenomenon I chose to call life review.* This review was healthy and psychologically powerful, but could have varied results, con-structive as well as anxiety-provoking and even terrifying. Among out-comes could be illumination of the self, perhaps its reinvention, atonement for regretted acts, redemption and forgiveness, and the possibility of recon-ciliation with family members or others where alienation existed. I searched the literature to discover whether anyone has used the term "life review" and I came up empty-handed.

I first reported this idea in an article "Recall and Retrospection" pub-lished in 1961. A more comprehensive article, "The Life Review—An inter-pretation of reminiscence in the aged" was published in 1963, since identi-fied as a "classic."

We all have stories, stories of our struggles through life, of our bonds and conflicts with our parents and siblings, spouses, children, friends, bosses, of our ups and downs, with laughter and tears, ambiguities, tri-umphs and defeats, and the comedies and tragedies of life, sometime [*sic*] writ large as national epics and odes. In the 17th century for the first time (with a few primitive exceptions) appeared autobiographies and memoirs—and novels, nearly always autobiographical.

I have looked back, too, and asked: "What leads a physician to gerontol-ogy?" A young practitioner did not find in his medical or clinical training in the 1950s—any more than today—much knowledge, sympathy or understanding of the mental and physical needs of the elderly, but my childhood compelled this interest.*

My grandparents reared me from infancy; [*sic*] my parents separated shortly after my birth, and when I was eleven months old, my mother brought me to live with her parents where my grandfather, then in his seventies, was a gentleman chicken farmer. I remember his blue overalls, his lined face and abundant white hair. He was my close friend and my teacher. Together we rose at 4 a.m. each day to feed the chickens, candle eggs, grow oats and tend to the sick chickens in the "hospital" at one end of the long chicken house. He would tell me of his younger days in Oklahoma and I would listen eagerly.

He disappeared suddenly when I was seven. I came back from a visit to a neighbor and he was gone. It made no sense. My grandmother said he went to visit relatives in Oklahoma—but he had not told me anything about the trip. With time, I realized I was never going to see him again. Dismay turned to fright and then to grief. I knew before they told me that he was dead.

Why? Why had he died? Why did people die? There was no talk, no funeral, only a "protective" silence that was more confusing than shared sorrow. I felt my silent way through a child's questions and a child's answers. Mostly, of course, I wanted to bring him back. Surely, someone could arrange it. Everyone ought to live forever. No, that clearly would make for too many problems: old people would accumulate in hordes and the world would be packed so tight there would be no room for babies.

Well, what about a commission to decide who should live and who should die? My grandfather would undoubtedly qualify for resurrection and continued life—but could I be certain the commission would recognize his special worth? Would there be cheating? Would there be mistakes? This did not appear to be a satisfactory answer either.

It was Dr. Rose, our white-haired family physician, who led me to a solution; I had cherished him for his reassuring presence and care through

*The following section is drawn from Butler's book, *Why Survive? Being Old in America* (1975).

my serious bout with scarlet fever. If Dr. Rose had been there with the right medicine, I would certainly have had my grandfather with me longer. To be a doctor was clearly the answer. For the first time my anxiety eased.

If love of my grandfather and old Dr. Rose brought me to medicine, it was my grandmother in the years that followed who showed me the strength and endurance of older persons. This was during the Depression. We lost the farm. She and I were soon on relief, eating government-surplus foods out of cans with stigmatizing white labels. My grandmother found work in a sewing room run by the WPA, and I sold newspapers and fixed bicycles for ten cents an hour. We moved into a hotel. When I was eleven, it burned to the ground with all our possessions. We started again. And what I remember even more than the hardships of those years was my grandmother's triumphant spirit and determination. Experiencing at first hand an older person's struggle to survive, I was myself helped to survive as well.

PART I: THE PAST

As I write it is also clear to me that I am already in the process of reviewing my own life, prompted by the realization of my own death, given the stage of my life, and by a few, happily only a few, imitations of morality. This has led me to better understand the goal of dealing with meaning in life cannot begin when one has been given a fatal or life-threatening diagnosis or is in one's death bed. Life review is a continuing process, reinforced at times of crisis in life and especially in the full realization of the finitude of life. But one can choose to review one's life earlier.

While the life review may emerge during many life crises, it is only the end of life, in old age, that one has the opportunity to look back on the entire life course. Schopenhauer wrote that "A complete and adequate notion of life can never be attained by anyone who does not reach old age; for it is only the old man who sees life whole and knows its natural course; it is only he who is acquainted—and this is the most important—not only with its entrance, like the rest of mankind, but with its exit too; so that he alone has a full sense of its utter vanity; whilst the others never cease to labor under the false notion that everything will come right in the end."

We inch along in our fifties and sixties, even seventies and eighties, only beginning to question what we have done and re-evaluating relationships. We may still make new commitments to ideas and people, to be re-evaluated in turn. As we grow still older and approach death, it becomes enormously important to strengthen our intimate relationships, to understand ourselves and our loved ones better, to come to grips with guilt and shame, experience remorse and serve others as well as effect reconciliations. We may come to confront and resolve acts of guilt by commission and omission through atonement and expiation. We may confess and seek forgiveness. Contrition can be sought. Note the tortured memoirs of Robert McNamara and François Mitterrand. The life review is not to be prettified. It is not peaches and cream. It must confront unresolved issues and dark negativisms. It can result in a serious depression, especially if done with help.

More influenced by Martin Buber than Erik Erikson, I have been especially impressed by the moral dimension attending "life reviews." In 1974 Myrna Lewis and I introduced "life review therapy" which is quite widely used, especially in homes for the aging, senior centers and elsewhere, by a variety of different specialists and in various countries in Asia and Europe.

But it is essential to know that life review is not an orderly process and that a series of sequential questions may not result in an evaluative life review. Life review is not simply a chronology but a passionate and evaluative, potentially life-enhancing but at times debilitating process. One is fortunate when one has empathic listeners who are either trained or uniquely gifted, and in an environment to be trusted. One needs a sense of privacy and to feel that one will not be embarrassed or assaulted in any way.

Reminiscence is the process of recollecting past experiences and events, or the experiences or events recollected. One-on-One and group reminiscence can be therapeutic but not evaluative, thereby distinguishing reminiscence from life review.

Life review is characterized by the progressive return to consciousness of past experiences and particularly, the resurgence of unresolved conflicts for reexamination and reintegration. If the reintegration is successful, such reminiscence can give new significance and meaning to life and prepare the person for death by mitigating fear and anxiety.

I believe this evaluative process occurs universally in all persons in the final years of their lives, although they may not be totally aware of it and may in part defend themselves against realizing its presence. It is spontaneous, unselective, and seen in other age groups as well especially when one is confronted by death or a major crisis; but the intensity and emphasis on putting one's life in order are most striking in old age. In late life, people have a particularly vivid imagination and memory for the past and can recall with sudden and remarkable clarity early life events. Individuals realize that their own personal myth of invulnerability and immortality can no longer be maintained. All of this results in reassessment of life, which, depending on the individual, may bring depression, acceptance or satisfaction.

The life review can occur in a mild form through mild nostalgia, mild regrets, a tendency to reminisce, tell stories, and the like. Often the life story will be told to anyone who will listen. At other times it is conducted in monologue in private, and is not meant to be overheard. It is in many ways similar to the psychotherapeutic situation in which a person is reviewing his or her life in order to understand present circumstances.

In severe forms the life review can lead to anxiety, guilt, despair and depression. And in extreme cases, if a person is unable to resolve problems or accept them, terror, panic and suicide can result. The most tragic life review is one in which the person decides that his/her life was a total waste.

Some of the positive results of a life review can be the righting of old wrongs, making up with enemies, coming to accept one's mortality, gaining a sense of serenity, pride in accomplishment and a feeling of having done one's best. Life review gives people an opportunity to decide what to do with the time left to them and work out emotional and material legacies. People become ready to die. The qualities of serenity and wisdom observable in some older people reflect a state of resolution of their life conflicts. This is usually accompanied by a lively capacity to live in the present, including the direct enjoyment of elemental pleasures such as nature, children, forms, colors, warmth, love and humor. Some become more capable of mutuality, with a comfortable acceptance of the life cycle, the universe and the generations. Creative works may result, such as memoirs, art, and music. People may put together family albums and scrapbooks and study their genealogies. It is useful to travel to one's birthplace and attend reunions.

There are life review and family history training manuals and guides to help people collect on audio- or videotape their life stories to leave to their families and others. Businesses have been created to sell audiotapes and videotapes and books made from interviews. Several aging organizations have developed material to help people create their own autobiographies or life reviews. In Britain, Age Exchange Reminiscence Centre has developed *A Practical Guide to Reminiscence.*

One of the great difficulties for younger persons (including mental health personnel) is to listen thoughtfully to the reminiscences of older people. Nostalgia is viewed as dysfunctional behavior, representative of living in the past, a preoccupation with self, as well as boring, meaningless, and time consuming. Yet, as a natural healing process, it represents one of the underlying human capacities on which all psychotherapy depends. The life review is a necessary and healthy process, and should be recognized in daily life as well as used in the mental health care of older people.

There have been a number of studies related to life review and life review therapy and there has been growing interest in related topics, such as storytelling, oral history, guided autobiography and narrative or experiential gerontology. The International Society of Reminiscence and Life Review was established in 1995.

Some writers take a dim view. "They live by memory rather than by hope, for what is left to them of life is but little compared to the long past. This, again, is the cause of their loquacity. They are continually talking of the past, because they enjoy remembering."—Aristotle in *Rhetoric* (367–347 BC).

"What makes old age hard to bear is not a failing of one's faculties, mental and physical, but the burden of one's memories."—Somerset Maugham in *Points of View* (1959).

Probably at no other time in life is there as potent a force toward self-awareness operating as in old age. Yet, the capacity to change, according to prevailing stereotype, decreases with age. "Learning capacity" falters with time, and it is fair to say that the major portion of gerontological research throughout the country is concerned almost enthusiastically with measuring decline in various cognitive, perceptual, and psychomotor functions.

In the course of the life review the older person may reveal to his wife, children, and other intimates, unknown qualities of his character and unstated actions of his past, as well as reveal heretofore undisclosed or unknown truths. Hidden themes of great vintage may emerge, changing the quality of a lifelong relationship. Revelations of the past may forge a new intimacy, render a deceit honest; they may sever peculiar bonds and free tongues; or they may sculpture terrifying hatreds or fluid fitful antagonisms.

• Ingmar Bergman's remarkable Swedish motion picture, *Wild Strawberries*, provides a beautiful example of the constructive aspects of the life review. Envisioning and dreaming of his past and his death, the protagonist-physician realizes the nonaffectionate and withholding qualities of his life; as the feeling of love reenters his life. The doctor changes even as death hovers upon him.

• One hospitalized 80-year-old woman, whose husband had died five years before had been discovered by her family berating her mirror image for her past deeds and shaking her fist at herself. She was preoccupied by past deeds and omissions in her personal relationships, as evidence [*sic*] by nursing notes.

• A 70-year-old woman communicated her concern with "God's wrath" and at various times gave intimations of her severe and intense sense of guilt about both past actions and past omissions. Her wish to kill herself seemed quite clear in both direct and indirect statements. Her past history strongly suggests she never realized her potentialities as a person and had never achieved an individual sense of identity. She was characterized by dependency, indecisiveness, self-centeredness, stubbornness, and a lack of generosity, despite the fact that she had stayed home to care for her mother and father after the other siblings had married. An attractive woman, she did not marry until a year and a half after her mother's death when she was 47.

• A 70-year-old retired and widowed mother came from another city to visit her son and showed no inclination to return home. Six months later, the son, anxious about his depressed, irritable mother, brought her to me.

She reluctantly accepted a psychotherapeutic relationship: Frightened and guarded, overly suspicious, she continually described her worthlessness; she considered herself so unworthy that she was not able to attend church. She was wrestling with guilt concerning past wrongs, acts both committed and avoided, and that she was afraid of death and judgment.

In one interview, she suddenly asked about privileged communication— that is, whether I would testify in a court of law against her if she were indicted for her past misdeeds. Later in the hour she said, "I am worried about my granddaughter—that something does not happen to her." She did not explain but added, "I wonder if she will be able to face her final examinations and graduation day." Since her granddaughter was an excellent student, she had little reason to worry. Still later in the hour she said, "My doctor referred to these black spots on my head as God's subpoenas." She was referring to brown, not black, senile freckles on her scalp. She went on to explain that she had been having difficulties getting her hair done properly and perhaps this was because she was contagious.

• Samuel Beckett's one-act play, *Krapp's Last Tape*, is a most compelling modern existential illustration of the life review. An old man listens uncomprehendingly to recordings he made as a young man in happier times. He is listening to a total stranger. The play asks, can he be regarded as the same human being in youth and old age?

Memories can involve all of the senses—taste, smell, vision, hearing, touch—and each may be exploited to evoke memories of the past. For Charles Dickens, for example, one whiff of a paste would bring back the anguish of his early years. Music is also a powerful stimulus for the flow of memories. The Hebrew Home for the Aged in New York City created in 1995 a lovely garden intended to trigger positive memories from the past. A porch swing evokes a bygone era, as does a water fountain made from a fire hydrant.

Remote memory is not as affected in the early stages of dementia as much as recent memory is. Life review and reminiscence techniques are used by nurses in nursing homes and as part of hospice care. The life review has been used in caring for terminally ill young adults with AIDS as well as older people. The National Hospice Foundation has used the concept of the life review and created a comprehensive guide for persons of all ages. Such a review should be available for those dying patients who wish to receive therapy that offers personal, existential, and spiritual help as well as palliative nursing and medicine.

THE VALIDITY OF THE LIFE REVIEW

Although the concept of the life review has become entrenched in both the literature and the practice of gerontology, nursing, social work, and to some degree psychology and psychiatry, aspects of the life review have been called into question, and many questions remain unanswered. For example, how does one determine whether memories have a factual basis or are defensive distortions? How effective or even possible is it to external verification of memories? Studies show, for example, that mothers' memories of the timing of the most simple events in their children's development, such as toilet training, are not always accurate. What are the interconnections between emotions and memories? Personal myths emerge from childhood and may be held throughout life, affecting one's self-image and most certainly influencing reminiscences. How do self-representations change over time? What is more important, that which is remembered or that which is forgotten, or both? How does one confirm findings that people regret most the things that they filed to do rather than the things they did do?

The life review helps both uncover and stabilize one's past selfhood. Tolstoy at age 81 said, "I remember very vividly that I am conscious of myself in exactly the same way now, at 81, as I was conscious of myself, my 'I' at five or six years of age." Consciousness is immovable. Due to this alone there is a movement that we call time. If time moves on, then there must be something that stands still; the consciousness of my "I" stand [sic] still. This is a common feeling, substantiated by extensive work at the National Institute on Aging's Baltimore Longitudinal Study of Aging.

Memory is a great force for human adaptation in general and is important to social evolution. The survival value of memory both to the individual and to society cannot be denied. Life review is important in itself; in a sense, it is analogous to undifferentiated, basic research. It adds to self-knowledge per se, independent of consequences. And, by extension, one learns of the lives of others and how lives might be led. As virtue is its own reward, so, too is the life review, for as Socrates said, "The unexamined life is not worth living." Put more positively, there are chances for pain, anger, guilt, and grief, but there are also opportunities for resolution and celebration, for affirmation and hope, for reconciliation and personal growth.

When a young person writes a novel he writes an autobiography; when an old personal writes an autobiography he writes a novel.

I believe "gentle closure," "peaceful death" or even a "good death" must mean dealing principally with the issues of life itself—the life one has led—and generally in the context of family, friends, and community. This is not an easy thing to do in the often impersonal, sterile, antiseptic medical atmosphere that we find in hospitals and nursing homes. In the cold Intensive Care Unit, kindness is almost subversive.

Note I did not disparage technology. I believe that technology, in fact, has enhanced the possibilities for a better death. We can harness technology and medications—to control pain, nausea, air hunger, and other symptoms. We need not be victimized by technology. Dying and death in past centuries was not so "tame," as the historian Philippe Aries would have us believe. We need to re-read biographies and history to remind ourselves and to understand how grim and painful dying and death could be and was so frequently. Now we also increasingly have the opportunity to create a kind of protocol for care at the end of life. Not a cookbook, but rather the goal would be to provide some degree of planning or negotiation so that people can die with increasingly full cognition and with needed time, given the technical capacity—to some degree—for the timing of death, with prospects of families being together. And reconciliation and forgiveness may be achieved in instances of strained and alienated relationships.

At what point would the physician or nurse give way to the rabbi, minster, priest or counselor? What are the responsibilities of the physician and the nurse beyond the realm of the body and its physical discomforts? Should the modern physician remain an *attending* physician in the best sense? To what degree can the nurse burdened by increasing administrative duties continue to serve?

Emotional, existential and spiritual care at end of life would be expected to be highly personal—and labor-intensive. While we know that the claimed high cost of dying is mythological, it may be that a truly effective end-of-life care program with gentle closure would be expensive unless we develop a volunteer program of well-trained individuals.

It is often said that America is a death-defying and death-denying culture. On the contrary, America seems to me to be obsessed with death and has been so from its historic violent beginnings, and we still have awesome violence in America. Our cinema and theater continue to document it. Denial, in fact, is a very useful and natural, even necessary defense, an important psychological phenomenon. It is universal, not particularly American. People should not and cannot be thinking about death all of the time. On the other hand, they cannot and should not avoid thinking about it either. Thus, a national conversation about death and dying is essential.

Much is made of the importance of having control and mastery over the end of one's life. Nietzsche said that the thought of suicide helps one get through many a difficult night. Suicide and/or physician-assisted suicide is reflected in public surveys as the ultimate control over one's self and one's death. This may be a contradiction, especially if influenced by subtle social and personal coercion. We must beware of the possibility that there can be public or family pressure for the patient to get out of the way.

We must also be careful that dying is not transformed into a narcissistic preoccupation, as exemplified in the statement "It is my own death and I must have control over it. It belongs to no one else!" Patient-controlled analgesia is one thing. Patient-controlled death which is *oblivious* to the needs of others is to be questioned. Is there not a family and community interest in our death by whatever means? Dying (and death) is not only a matter of one's own personhood. It must be seen in a larger social context. That is true of death in general and perhaps suicide in particular. Death leaves profound effects upon those left behind, the bereaved. Suicide may reverberate down a number of generations as we so often see clinically. In a sense, one's choice of the form of death is perceived, however correctly or incorrectly, as the value that one places upon life. Albert Camus felt that the question of suicide was the essential philosophic question.

Data have shown that one-fifth of the world's people do not list a religious affiliation or belief. They are apparently agnostic, atheistic or hold idiosyncratic views, separate from organized religions. Apparently millions do not believe in an after-life, and do not believe in organized religion. But they often feel intimidated by the larger society in which they live, especially in these times of rising fundamentalism in Christianity and Islam. Disbelievers are not in favor. On the other hand, Paul Tillich suggested that agnostics may be next to God since, in his view, they struggle so much. There are numerous atheists in foxholes. There is no compelling evidence that one's religious attitude affects the nature of one's death. Death, like life, benefits from freedom of thought.

There are great responsibilities that must be placed upon and accepted by those of us entrusted with the precious and very special moments of life that follow disease and end in dying and death. Once physicians and priests, for example, were one and the same (e.g., the shaman) and often were thought to be supernatural or charismatic. Some were also leaders of their tribes. Those who led us through the valley of the shadow of death have the responsibility to help us deal with disillusion and help us hold a vision of the larger world that links us with others and with the universe.

PART II: THE PRESENT

Jung wrote in *Modern Man in Search of a Soul*, "We cannot live the afternoon of life according to the program of life's morning, for what was great in the morning will be little at evening, and what in the morning was true, will at evening have become a lie. I have given psychological treatment to too many people of advancing years, and have looked too often into the secret chambers of their souls, not to be moved by this fundamental truth. . . . "

"Especially at this moment, when I perceive that my life is so brief in time, I try to increase it in weight; I try to arrest the speed of its flight by the speed with which I grasp it, and compensate for the haste of its ebb by my vigor in using it. The shorter my possession of life, the deeper and fuller I must make it," wrote Michel Montaigne.

"Some sigh for yesterday. Some for tomorrow! But you must reach old age before you can understand the meaning—splendid, absolute, unchallengeable, irreplaceable meaning—of the word 'today,' " said Paul Claudel.

Illustrations:

- Joyce Cary's novel *To Be a Pilgrim* about old age describes vividly recollections of long past rain against a window pane and a sister's delighted laughter.
- A story by Solzhenitsyn of a prisoner in the gulag who comes to experience his full being with the wet grass under his feet.
- A diary entry of the art historian Bernard Berenson in *Sunset and Twilight* who in his 90's feels he now sees for the first time the colors and geometry of the Tuscan hills as the Renaissance painters experienced them—freed from the "barnacles of scholarship," quoting him.
- Victor Frankl in *From Death Camp to Existentialism* discovers the life-saving aspects of focusing on the immediate limited choices available to him in a concentration camp.

Fears about time running out may be reduced and replaced with a sense of immediacy, or the here and now. The elemental things in life—children, friendship, nature, human touching (physical and emotional), colors, shapes—gain significance as people sort out the more important things in life from the less important. Recall the common Anglo Saxon roots for the words holy, healthy and healing. Perhaps elementality bears some relationship with the Eastern contemplative tradition.

Sense of Presentness and Immediacy

John Bayley refers to the Reverend Sydney Smith who "used to urge parishioners in the grip of depression . . . to take short views of human life—never further than dinner or tea" (Bayley, John. *Elegy For Iris*, St. Martin's Press, 1998). This advice illustrates the therapeutic use of "presentness."

We wish a particular day's work were done, even that a vacation were over. Why do we wish our life away? What strange compulsion is this? We often blend our present with the future, and our preoccupation with the future often overwhelms the present. Consequently, we do not fully enjoy the present. This continuing pull of the future is not easily explained. Why do we have so much trouble enjoying the moment? This was not as true when we were children.

Older persons often rediscover the capacity to enjoy the fullness of the moment. The recovery of the present is a kind of rediscovery of childhood. I call this internalization of the moment *elementality* or *presentness*. It encompasses an emotional vocabulary of pleasure. Elementality demonstrates the beneficence of nature. Much of mankind has become separated from the soil. Men and women of the industrialized world no longer use their own hands to grow things, or hunt and fish. This blunt separation from nature carries a severe punishment, in that we lose important elemental aspects of human existence and survival. Over time, there emerges a layered accumulation of psychological, social, historical and theological influences that reduces our relationship with nature. Elementality is often replaced by ambition which, when successful, assumes power. Can we strip layers away? Can we give up power? The so-called mellowing with age may be the happy consequence of recovered elementality.

In elementality, one finds the early outlines of life may be far richer than the complicated lifetime of experiences, images and defenses that cover it up. There is a dark side to the lives of those of wealth and privilege; they do not need to carry out the most elemental aspects of existence, the preparing of their own food and taking care of their own personal needs. In a perverse sense, elementality is a luxury of poverty.

There may be a resolution of time panics ("time running out") and boredom and there may be a more appropriate valuation of time. By middle age we begin to be concerned with the number of years left to life. The elemental things of life such as children, friendship, human touching (physical and emotional), colors and shapes assume greater significance as people sort out the more important from the less important. Simple pleasure comes from breathing in the air, tasting the water and chewing food. The pre-Spring appearance of snowdrops is a cause for celebration. This is a revitalization, a return to the spontaneity of childhood and its pleasures. Old age can become a time of emotional and sensory awareness and enjoyment. Elementality helps define wisdom. One way to experience elementality is to recover specific memories and emotions such as the afternoon glow of a summer's day, an electric storm, a cool fall evening, a mother's hand against a feverish forehead or the love of flowers in springtime. When we recover such memories of a distant childhood, we gain strength and a sense of peace. Elementality, pensive and evocative, is a way to freedom from anxiety.

Elementality or presentness takes us back to preverbal mechanisms and transitional objects, such as the comfort of a teddy bear, that carries us from the protection of a mother to the reality of the outer world. Olfactory memories, such as Vicks vapor rub or a mustard pad, to simple tactile maneuvers like kissing and "making better" the scrapped knee unite the past with the present.

In a healthy family, in childhood, one is relatively anxiety-free and life is pleasurable, *before time and anxiety are discovered*. When the child discovers prolonged separation or death, anxiety enters and elementality lessens. With the recognition of death comes an awareness of a past and anticipation of a future. Throughout life we sometimes recapture a sense of elementality when we discover that we do not know "where the time went" while we were enjoying life, either at work or on vacation, temporarily free of anxiety.

We are *not* referring to "second childhood," a banal and ageist notion, suggestive of regression, and pathology. Nor does elementality refer to the normal, natural re-creation of certain elements of the past. However, there is a "second childhood" that is rich with meaning and not always achieved—the recovery of the emotional texture of the beginnings of one's life.

Old age has a limited future, with a fading—but not elimination—of dreams and opportunities. Upon his return to _____ [*sic*] after his space flight at 77, John Glenn said, "Old men can have dreams too." One of the tasks of late life is learning not to think as much in terms of the future but to confront and deal with the past, and to live to the fullest in the moment, emphasizing the quality of the time remaining rather than the quantity.

Mortimer J. Adler, the philosopher, echoing Plato, wrote, "The young can be prepared for education in the years to come, but only mature men and women can become educated—beginning the process in their forties and fifties and reaching some modicum of genuine insight, sound judgment and practical wisdom after they have turned 60." An educated person is one who has assimilated the ideas that make him representative of his culture, a bearer of his traditions, and one who continues to learn. There is a cartoon at an _____ [sic] by Goya—Goya with the caption "I am still learning."

Older people are returning to school in droves—Elderhostel in the U.S. and the Third Age universities in France. Genealogy-tourism, family vacations, eco-tourism, study tours and holidays to the museums and monuments, and learning languages are popular, too. Information technology is among the most selected courses. Eighty-year-olds, owning personal computers, are on the Internet.

Bernard Berenson's descriptions of "life-enhancing experiences" are characterized as spontaneous, elusive, natural and simple rather than artificial and elaborate. Berenson spoke of "making life a work of art." This requires work, not wasting time on non-essentials and learning to say "no." It offers still the opportunity for a sensuous appreciation of life.

It is as if we see a *new stage of life* unfolding. Old age is no longer equivalent to disease, infirmity, frailty, decrepitude and slowing down. The brain is proving to be subject to repair and growth and this plasticity promises greater cognitive health.

Some evident characteristics of late life are markedly reinforced, such as the desire to leave a mark, by sponsoring and mentoring, by philanthropy and volunteering; by reminiscence and reflection, now more commonly welcomed, and *even by rebellion that follows the freedom from the need to earn one's daily bread.*

Maggie Kuhn said, "When I turned 80, I made a resolution to do something outrageous every week—which I kept up until recently. Now I try to do something outrageous every day."

But, with the new rich stage of life come new responsibilities and new obligations. New roles and different conception of age regarding work and citizenship advance the human condition. The challenge is how to better understand, shape and value this new old age. Older persons themselves should *define this portion of their lives*, and not passively allow the culture to do so. They are the pioneers who have entered into this redefined old age and do not accept aging and disability as inevitable, unpreventable and untreatable. Society and culture, of course, have catching up to do.

Quetelet's search for the "average man" is probably hopeless. Life is messy and not rigidly scheduled, and milestones and timelines are not faultlessly set on automatic. Choices and dilemmas abound. The destination is never clear, the goals never entirely met. Hopes are dashed, hurts pile up, unexpected connections are riveted together, strength builds in the face of challenges and surprises constantly await. Quetelet notwithstanding, the outline of life is more drama than systematic regularity, and life's odyssey—the drama of life—is infinitely more exciting and mysterious.

Michel de Montaigne [wrote], "I speak truth, not so much as I would, but as much as I dare; and I dare more as I grow older." And Leo Tolstoy made clear "Old age is the most unexpected of all things that happen to a man." Pindar in the Olympiads (5th century) wisely said, "Do not yearn after immortality, but exhaust the limits of the possible."

PART III: TRANSITIONS

I gave a testimony before the Senate Health, Education, Labor and Pensions (HELP) Committee on January 26, 2009. I spoke of healthy aging.

Healthy aging of course requires a life span perspective. We must engage the public to remain vigorous and healthy throughout life. In a sense, we all know what we need to do, but it is just very hard to do it. The seven key needs are:

1. Physical exercise
2. Appropriate low caloric diet
3. Minimal alcohol
4. No smoking
5. Efforts against stress reduction and management
6. Having a strong social network and support system, intimacy and love
7. Having a sense of dedicated purpose

We know that prospects for developing health promotion and disease prevention is [sic] far beyond the possibilities of the doctor-patient relationship. Doctors today have no longer than 12 minutes to see a patient. We must therefore undertake a public health perspective following the model of tobacco and alcohol beverages through added taxation and education. There should be modernization of the 15,000 senior centers in the United States to promote health and encourage the contributions of older people to their communities. Finally, we need a national walking movement to get people walking together, friends, neighbors, families. This is an inexpensive way to help overcome the serious growth of obesity in America.

People not only want to simply live long, but to remain in good healthy. We pretty much know the necessary ingredients, but it is very difficult to live up to the requirements.

The seven key features of healthy aging are:

1. Appropriate low caloric diet with 7–9 fruits and vegetables each day, multivitamins in particular vitamin D (with sunlight to activate vitamin D).

2. Physical activity including (1) aerobics, that is reasonably strenuous walk five days a week; (2) muscle strengthening, particularly of the quadriceps or thigh muscle, through squats. It is known that the quadriceps is the primary predictor of frailty in old age. Falls is the number twelve cause of death for people over 65 and muscle strength and balance are critical; (3) balance; (4) flexibility; (5) posture.

3. Smoking cessation

4. Moderate use of alcohol, the equivalent of no more than one glass of wine per day.

5. Managing stress, most difficult of all efforts though medication, yoga, visualization, mini vacations and appropriate sleep.

6. Building a strong support system and social network of friends and relationships, especially intimacy and love. This may be one reason why women outlive men, because they have a stronger capacity for dealing with intimacy.

7. A sense of purpose—something to get up for in the morning. We discovered in studies we did at the National Institutes of Health back in the 1950s and 60s that those individuals that had something to get up for in the morning, something purposeful, lived longer and better.

We know that perhaps no more than 25% of our health and longevity depends upon genes. Thus some 75% is up to us. This offers us a lot of power, but also entails genuine responsibility of self care.

Taxation and education were very effective in the 50% reduction of smokers in the United States since 1964. On the other hand, alcohol in America is marked by a significant number of hard core alcoholics affecting one of every four American families, accounting for most domestic abuse and a significant contribution to highway fatalities and other accidents. Alcohol taxes used to constitute a significant part of Federal revenue. In fact, there have been only a few increases in liquor taxes since 1950. This is an issue that should be revisited by Congress.

Citizens of America, the President's Council on Physical Fitness and Sports, the U.S. Prevention Task Forces and other appropriate organizations should sponsor a national walking movement. This is not expensive and it does not require membership in a health club.

Of course healthy aging is a life course issue, it is not something you simply introduce at fifty, sixty or beyond. A few years ago, several of us wrote a widely quoted paper in the *New England Journal of Medicine* on the problem of obesity in America and the prospect that we might lose 3 to 5 years of life expectancy from the thirty additional years of life we gained in the 20th century. Further, for the first time in our history, our children might live less long than their parents. It is quite terrible to see 10 year old children who are obese and who already have type two old age diabetes.

Frailty

Dementia

As the end of life approaches, there is a loss of the ability to project into the future, an observation made in the 1950s by Eduardo Krapf, Argentinean psychoanalyst.

THE FUTURE

Starting over is one of the prospects of later life, a second career in a changing society. There is ReServe, the Experience Corps and other nonprofit, non-governmental opportunities, careers that have a larger social impact—in education, healthcare, government, non-profits.

REFERENCES

Abbott, A. 1988. *The System of Professions: An Essay on the Division of Expert Labor.* Chicago: University of Chicago Press.

Achenbaum, W. A. 1978. *Old Age in the New Land: The American Experience Since 1790.* Baltimore: Johns Hopkins University Press.

———. 1986. *Social Security: Visions and Revisions.* New York: Cambridge University Press.

———. 1995. *Crossing Frontiers: Gerontology Emerges as a Science.* New York: Cambridge University Press.

———. 2005. *Older Americans, Vital Communities: A Bold Vision for Societal Aging.* Baltimore: Johns Hopkins University Press.

———. 2010. "Gene D. Cohen, MD, PhD: Creative Gero-Psychiatrist and Visionary Public Intellectual." *Journal of Aging, Humanities, and Arts* 4 (December): 238–50.

———. 2012. *How Boomers Turned Conventional Wisdom on Its Head.* White Paper. Westport, Conn.: MetLife Mature Market Institute.

Achenbaum, W. A., and D. M. Albert. 1995. *Profiles in Gerontology: A Biographical Dictionary.* Westport, Conn.: Greenwood Press.

Adelman, R. C. 1995. "The Alzheimerization of Aging." *Gerontologist* 35 (4): 526–32.

"Aging Well." 2008. *Q & A with Robert N. Butler* 1 (2): 42. http://www.agingwellmag
.com/archive/spring08p42.shtml.

Alliance for Aging Research (AAR). 2001. *The Legendary Lifetime of Senator Alan
Macgregor Cranston.* http://agingresearch.org/content/article/detail/910.

Alliance Trends Resources. n.d. *Aged and Eldercare.* http://www.alliancetrends
.org/resources.cfm?id=91.

Altbach, P. G., R. O. Berdahl, and P. J. Gumport, eds. 2005. *American Higher Education in the Twenty-First Century.* 2d ed. Baltimore: Johns Hopkins University Press.

Amazon.com. n.d. *Why Survive?* http://www.amazon.com/Why-Survive-Being
-Old-America/dp/0801874254/ref=sr_1_1?ie=UTF8&qid=1343449943&sr=8
-1&keywords=why+survive+being+old+in+America.

American Board of Medical Specialties (ABMS). n.d. *Who We Are and What We
Do.* http://www.abms.org/ about_abms/who_we_are.aspx.

American Federation for Aging Research. n.d. Links. http://www.afar.org/media
/links.

American Medical Association (AMA). 1959. *Archives of General Psychiatry* 1 (6).

Anlyan, W. G., and J. Graves. 1973. *The Future of Medical Education.* Durham:
Duke University Press.

Anton-Luca, A. 1998. "Anthropologist Biographies: Gregory Bateson (1904–1980)."
http://www.indiana.edu/~wanthro/theory_pages/Bateson.htm.

Arnst, C. 2007. "Decoding Alzheimer's." *BusinessWeek.*

Atchley, R. C. 1983. *Aging: Continuity and Change.* Belmont, Calif.: Wadsworth.

Baker, G. T., and R. L. Sprott. 1988. "Biomarkers of Aging." *Experimental Gerontology* 23 (4–5): 223–39.

Ballenger, J. F. 2006. *Self, Senility, and Alzheimer's Disease in Modern America.*
Baltimore: Johns Hopkins University Press.

Baltes, P. B. 2003. "Extending Longevity: Dignity Gain—or Dignity Drain." *Aging
Research* (March): 15–19.

Baltes, P. B., and K. U. Mayer. 2001. *The Berlin Aging Study.* New York: Cambridge
University Press.

Baltes, P. B., and J. Smith. 2003. "New Frontiers in the Future of Aging: From Successful Aging of the Young Old to the Dilemmas of the Fourth Age." *Gerontology* 49:123–35.

Baranauckas, C. 2002. "Florence S. Mahoney, 103, Health Advocate." *New York
Times.* December 16. http://www.nytimes.com/2002/12/16/us/florence-s
-mahoney-103-health-advocate.html.

"Barbara Walters Has a New Man." n.d. *Insider.* http://www.theinsider.com
/news/126378_Barbara_Walters_Has_A_New_Man.

Barfield, C. E. 1982. *Science Policy from Ford to Reagan.* Washington, D.C.: American Enterprise Institute.

Barondes, S. H. 1990. "The Biological Approach to Psychiatry: History and Prospects." *Journal of Neuroscience* 10:1707–10.

Bartels, S. J., F. C. Blow, L. M. Brockman, and A. D. van Citters. 2005. *Substance Abuse and Mental Health Among Older Americans.* Rockville, Md.: WESTAT.

Barzun, J. 1947. *Teacher in America.* Boston: Little, Brown.

Bauerlein, M. 2010. "21st-Century Public Intellectuals." *Chronicle of Higher Education.*

Beam, A. 2008. *A Great Idea at the Time.* New York: Public Affairs.

Bearn, A. G. 1978. "Robert Frederick Loeb: March 14, 1895–October 21, 1973." In *Biographical Memoirs.* Vol. 85. Washington, D.C.: National Academies Press.

Beck, J. C., and R. N. Butler. 2004. "Physician Recruitment into Geriatrics— Further Insight into the Black Box." *Journal of the American Geriatrics Society* 52:1959–61.

Beeson, P. B. 1985. "The Institute of Medicine Report on Aging and Medical Education: 1984 Update." *Bulletin of the New York Academy of Medicine* 61:478–83.

Bell, D. 1966. *The Reforming of General Education: The Columbia Experience in Its National Setting.* New York: Columbia University Press.

———. 1980. *The Winding Passage.* Cambridge: Abt Books.

Benen, S. 2011. "America: Dumbing Down . . . Down . . . Down." *All Things Wildly Considered.* January 25. http://allthingswildlyconsidered.blogspot.com/2011/01 /america-dumbing-downdowndown.html.

Bennett, Ronni. 2011. "The Best Books on Aging." *Time Goes By.* http://www .timegoesby.net/weblog/the-best-books-on-aging.html.

Bensing, K. 2008. "Q&A: Robert Butler." *Library Journal.* February 1. http://www .libraryjournal.com/article/CA6524666.html?q=robert+n . . .

Berger, A., B. J. Small, Y. Forsell, B. Winblad, and L. Backman. 1998. "Preclinical Symptoms of Major Depression in Very Old Age." *American Journal of Psychiatry* 155:1039–43.

Berkman, B. 1978. "Mental Health and the Aging: A Review of the Literature for Clinical Social Workers." *Clinical Social Work* 6:230–45.

Berliner, R. W., and T. J. Kennedy. 1970. "National Expenditures for Biomedical Research." *Journal of Medical Education* 45:666–78.

Bernard, M. A., P. Blanchette, and K. Brummel-Smith. 2009. "Strength and Influence of Geriatrics Departments in American Health Centers." *Academic Medicine* 84:627–32.

Bernstein, C. 1969. "Age and Race Fears Seen in Housing Opposition." *Washington Post.* March 7.

Binstock, R. H. 2003. "The War on 'Anti-Aging Medicine.'" *Gerontologist* 43:4–14.

Birren, J. E., and D. E. Deutchman. 1991. *Guiding Autobiography Groups for Older Adults.* Baltimore: Johns Hopkins University Press.

Birren, J. E., R. N. Butler, S. W. Greenhouse, L. Sokoloff, and M. R. Yarrow, eds. 1963. *Human Aging: A Biological and Behavioral Study.* Bethesda, Md.: National Institute of Health.

Birren, J. E., et al. 1996. *Aging and Biography.* New York: Springer.

Blankenhorn, D. 2010. "The Man Who Transformed Aging and Death, at Peace." *Smartplanet.* July 7. http://www.smartplanet.com/technology/blog/rethinking-healthcare/the-man-who-transformed-aging-and-death-at-peace/1376.

Bobbio, N. 2001. *Old Age and Other Essays.* Translated by Allan Cameron. Cambridge, UK: Polity.

Bodenheimer, T. 2006. "Primary Care—Will It Survive?" *New England Journal of Medicine* 355:861–64.

Bohlmeijer, E. T., and G. J. Westerhof. 2010. *Storying One's Life: Your Autobiography as a Source of Wisdom.* Amsterdam: Uitgeverij Boom.

Bohlmeijer, E. T., G. J. Westerhof, and M. Emmerik de-Jong. 2008. "The Effects of Integrative Reminiscence on Meaning in Life." *Aging and Mental Health* 12:302–4.

Booth, W., comp. 1992. *The Art of Growing Older.* New York: Poseidon Press.

Bornstein, M. B. 1989. "In Memoriam: Margaret Ransone Murray." *Journal of Neuropathology and Experimental Neurology* 48 (1): 111–12.

Bortz, W. M. 2007. *We Live Too Short and Die Too Long.* New York: SelectBooks.

Bowers, J. Z. 1978. "Willard Cole Rappleye (1892–1976)." *Bulletin of the New York Academy of Medicine* 54:879–80.

Bowman, K. M. 1939. "The Modern Treatment of Schizophrenia." *Bulletin of the New York Academy of Medicine* 15 (May): 338–53.

Bowman, K. M., and A. Simon. 1948. "Studies in Electronarcosis Therapy." *American Journal of Psychiatry* 105:15–27.

Bowman, K. M., A. Simon, C. H. Hine, E. A. Macklin, G. H. Crook, N. Burbridge, and K. A. Hanson. 1951. "Clinical Evaluation of Tetraethylthiuramdisulphide (Antabuse) in the Treatment of Problem Drinkers." *American Journal of Psychiatry* 107:832–38.

Boyd, R. R., and C. G. Oakes, eds. 1973. *Foundations of Practical Gerontology.* Columbia: University of South Carolina Press.

Boydston, J. A., ed. 1986. *John Dewey: The Later Works.* Vol. 9. Carbondale: Southern Illinois University Press.

Boynton, R. S. 1991. "Princeton's Public Intellectual: A Profile of Cornel West." *New York Times Magazine.* September 15. http://www.nytimes.com/1991/09/15 /magazine/princeton-s-public-intellectual.html.

Bramwell, A. 2010. "Not Even Joseph Epstein Speaks Freely About the Conservative Movement." *League of Ordinary Gentlemen.* http://ordinary-gentlemen .com/blog/2010/07/03/not-even-joseph-epstein-speaks-freely-about-the-conser vative-movement

Brandt, A. M. 1987. *No Magic Bullet.* New York: Oxford University Press.

Brekke, J. S., K. Eli, and L. A. Palinkas. 2007. "Translational Science at the National Institute of Mental Health: Can Social Work Take Its Rightful Place?" *Research on Social Work Practice* 17:123–33.

Brennan, E. A., and E. C. Clarage. 1999. *Who's Who of Pulitzer Prize Winners.* Phoenix: Oryx Press.

Brody, J. A., J. Cornoni-Huntley, and C. H. Patrick. 1981. "Research Epidemiology as a Growth Industry at the National Institute on Aging." *Public Health Reports* 96:269–73.

Brown, E. 2010. "Father of Modern Gerontology Robert N. Butler Dies at 83." *Washington Post.* July 7.

Brown, J. F. 1940. "Freud's Influence on American Psychology." *Psychoanalytic Quarterly* 9:283–92.

Brumfiel, G. 2008. "Older Scientists Publish More Papers." *Nature* 455:1161.

Brunton, L., L. Goodman, J. Lazo, A. Gilman, and K. Parker, eds. 2006. *Goodman & Gilman's The Pharmacological Basis of Therapeutics.* New York: McGraw-Hill.

Buck, P. H., J. Finley, R. Demos, L. Hoadley, B. S. Hollinshead, W. Jordan, and B. F. Wright. 1945. *General Education in a Free Society.* Cambridge: Harvard University Press.

Bullard, D. M., H. H. Glaser, M. C. Heagarty, and E. C. Pivchik. 1967. "Failure to Thrive in the 'Neglected' Child." *American Journal of Orthopsychiatry* 37:680–90.

Burger, W. R. 2008. *Human Services in Contemporary America.* 7th ed. Belmont, Calif.: Brookes-Cole.

Burnett, B. 2009. "The Dumbing of America." *Huffington Post.com.* October 16. http:// www.huffingtonpost.com/bob-burnett/the-dumbing-of-america_b_323528.html.

Bury, C. ca. 2005. "Collington History." http://www.keepingupwithcollington.org /Collington%20History.htm.

Bush, V. 1946. *Endless Horizons.* Washington, D.C.: Public Affairs Press.

Busse, E. W., R. H. Barnes, A. J. Silverman, G. M. Shy, M. Thaler, and L. L. Frost. 1954. "Studies of the Process of Aging: Factors That Influence the Psyche of Elderly Persons." *American Journal of Psychiatry* 110:897–903.

Butler, R. N. 1960. "Intensive Psychotherapy for the Hospitalized Aged. *Geriatrics* 15:644–53.

———. 1961. "Re-awakening Interests." *Nursing Homes: Journal of the American Nursing Home Association* 10:8–19.

———. 1963a "Privileged communication and confidentiality in research." *Archives of General Psychiatry* 8:139–41.

———. 1963b. "The Life Review: An Interpretation of Reminiscence in the Aged." *Psychiatry* 26:65–76.

———. 1967. "Aspects of Survival and Adaptation in Human Aging." *American Journal of Psychiatry* 123:1233–43.

———. 1969a. "The Burnt-Out and the Bored." *Washington Monthly* 1:58–60.

———. 1969b. "The Effects of Medical and Health Progress on the Social and Economic Aspects of the Life Cycle." *Industrial Gerontology* 2:1–9.

———. 1970. "Guest Editorial: Immediate and Long-range Dangers to Transfer of Elderly Patients from State Hospitals to Community Facilities." *Gerontologist* 10:259–60.

———. 1971a. "The Public Interest Report No. 1." *International Journal of Aging and Human Development* 2:139–41.

———. 1971b. "The Public Interest Report No. 2: Old Age in Your Nation's Capital." *International Journal of Aging and Human Development* 2:197–201.

———. 1974. "Successful Aging and the Role of the Life Review." *Journal of the American Geriatrics Society*, 529–35.

———. 1975a. "Psychiatry and the Elderly: An Overview." *American Journal of Psychiatry* 132:893–900.

———. 1975b. *Why Survive? Being Old in America*. New York: Harper & Row.

———. 1976. "Guest Editorial: Early Directions for the National Institute on Aging." *Gerontologist* 16:293–94.

———. 1979. "Geriatrics and Internal Medicine." *Annals of Internal Medicine* 91:903–8.

———. 1980. "Collaboration Between National Institutes of Gerontology: Actual and Potential." Meeting of Directors of National Institutes of Gerontology in Weimar, Germany, October 20–21. Washington, D.C.: World Health Organization.

———. 1981. "The Teaching Nursing Home." *Journal of the American Medical Association* 245:1435–37.

———. 1982. "Charting the Conquest of Senility." *Bulletin of the New York Academy of Medicine* 58:362–81.

———. 1983a. "The Relation of Extended Life to Extended Employment Since the Passage of Social Security in 1935." *Milbank Fund Quarterly* 61:420–29.

———. 1983b. Interview by J. Caldwell [Audio Tape Recording]. "An Interview with Robert Butler." *Gerontologist* 23:8–12.

———. 1983c. "An Overview of Research on Aging and the Status of Gerontology Today." *Milbank Memorial Quarterly* 61 (Summer): 351.

———. 1984. *A Generation at Risk: When the Baby Boomers Reach Golden Pond.* Austin: Hogg Foundation for Mental Health.

———. 1985. "Summary Remarks—Geriatric Medical Education Imperative." *Bulletin of the New York Academy of Medicine* 61:665–72.

———. 1987. "Foreword." In *Modern Biological Theories of Aging.* Edited by H. R. Warner, R. N. Butler, R. L. Sprott, and E. L. Schneider. New York: Raven Press.

———. 1990. "The Contributions of Late Life Creativity to Society." *Gerontology & Geriatrics Education* 11:45–52.

———. 1993a. "The Importance of Basic Research in Gerontology." *Age and Ageing* 22 (Sup. 1): S53–S54.

———. 1993b. "Japan and U.S. Health Policies for the 21st Century: The Role of Geriatrics." *Japan and the World Economy* 5:157–71.

———. 1994. "Introduction." In *Productive Aging and the Role of Older People in Japan: New Approaches for the United States.* By S. A. Bass. New York: Japan Society and International Longevity Center.

———. 1996. Foreword to *Hannah's Heirs.* By D. A. Pollen. New York: Oxford University Press.

———. 1998a. "John Glenn: Star Trek II." *Geriatrics* 53:17–18.

———. 1998b. "Presentation to the National Bipartisan Commission on the Future of Medicare." April 20. http://thomas.loc.gov/medicare/butler_test.html.

———. 1999. "Is the National Institute on Aging Mission Out of Balance?" *Gerontologist* 39:389–91.

———. 2002a. "Declaration of the Rights of Older Persons." United Nations Second World Assembly on Ageing, NFO World Forum on Ageing. New York: International Longevity Center.

———. 2002b. "Life Review." In *Encyclopedia on Aging.* http://www.encyclopedia.com/doc/lG2–3402200232.html.

———. 2003a. "Executive Summary." In *Longevity Genes: From Primitive Organisms to Humans.* Edited by H. R. Warner. New York: International Longevity Center.

———. 2003b. "Selected as the Best Paper in JAGS in the 1970s: Mission of the National Institute on Aging." *Journal of the American Geriatrics Society* 51 (8): 1169–73.

———. 2005a. "Do Longevity and Health Generate Wealth?" *Cambridge Handbook of Age and Ageing.* Edited by M. L. Johnson, V. L. Bengtson, and P. Coleman, 546–51. Cambridge: Cambridge University Press.

———. 2005b. "Foreword." In *Encyclopedia of Ageism.* Edited by E. B. Palmore, L. Branch, and D. K. Harris. New York: Haworth Press.

———. 2005c. "Ageism: Looking Back Over My Shoulder." *Generations* 29 (Fall): 84–86.

———. 2006. *Ageism in America.* New York: International Longevity Center USA.

———. 2007. "Thoughts on the Development of Geriatrics." *Journal of the American Geriatrics Society* 55:2086–87.

———. 2008. *The Longevity Revolution: The Benefits and Challenges of Living a Long Life.* New York: Public Affairs.

———. 2009. "Combating Ageism." *International Psychogeriatrics* 21:211.

———. 2010a. *The Longevity Prescription: The 8 Proven Keys to a Long, Healthy Life.* New York: Avery/Penguin Group.

———. 2010b. "Prologue or Introduction to Life Review." Mss.

———. n.d. "Memorandum of Understanding to Mt. Sinai."

Butler, R. N., D. K. Dastor, and S. Perlin. 1965. "Relationships of Senile Manifestations and Chronic Brain Syndromes to Cerebral Circulation and Metabolism." *Journal of Psychiatric Research* 3:229–38.

Butler, R. N., and H. P. Gleason, eds. 1985. "Introduction." In *Productive Aging: Enhancing Vitality in Later Life.* New York: Springer.

Butler, R. N., and C. Jasmin. 2000. *Longevity and Quality of Life.* New York: Kluwer Academic/Plenum.

Butler, R. N., and K. Kiikuni. 1993. *Who Is Responsible for My Old Age?* New York: Springer.

Butler, R. N., and M. I. Lewis. 1976. *Sex After Sixty: A Guide for Men and Women for Their Lateral Years.* New York: Harper and Row.

———. 1982. *Aging and Mental Health: Positive Psychosocial Approaches.* 3d ed. St. Louis: C. V. Mosby.

———. 1988. *Midlife Love Life: How to Deal with the Physical and Emotional Changes of Midlife and Their Effect on Your Sex Life.* New York: HarperCollins.

Butler, R. N., and M. M. Osako. 1990. "Planning for Old Age: How Japan Is Looking Ahead." *Washington Post Health* 6.

Butler, R. N., and L. G. Sullivan. 1963. "Psychiatric Contact with the Community-Resident, Emotionally Disturbed Elderly." *Journal of Nervous and Mental Disease* 137:180–86.

Butler, R. N., H. R. Warner, T. F. Williams, S. N. Austad, J. A. Brody, J. Campisi, J., and W. E. Write. 2003. "The Aging Factor in Health and Disease: The Promise of Basic Research on Aging." *Aging Clinical and Experimental Research* 16:104–11.

Bytheway, B. 2005. "Ageism and Age Characterization." *Journal of Social Issues* 61:361–74.

Cahan, R. B., and C. L. Yeager. 1967. "Admission EEG as a Predictor of Mortality and Discharge for Aged State Hospital Patients." *Journal of Gerontology* 21:248–56.

Califano, J. A. 1979. "The Government-Medical Education Partnership." *Journal of Medical Education* 54:19.

Campbell, M. L. 1993. "Aging with a Disability: A Life Course Perspective." http://codi.buffalo.edu.graph_based_aging/conf/.life.htm.

Cappella, J. N., and K. H. Jamieson. 1997. *Spiral of Cynicism: The Press and the Public Good.* New York: Oxford University Press.

Cappeliez, P. 2002. "Cognitive-Reminiscence Therapy for Depressed Older Adults in Day Hospital and Long-term Care." In *Critical Advances in Reminiscence Work.* Edited by J. Webster and B. Haight. New York: Springer.

Carleton, W. 1873. "Over the Hill to the Poor-house." In *Farm Ballads.* New York: Harper & Brothers.

Carlson, M. 2010. "Robert Butler Obituary." *Guardian* (UK). July 18.

Carlyle, T. 1888. *On Heroes, Hero-Worship and the Heroic in History.* New York: Frederick A. Stokes.

Carstensen, L. 2009. *A Long Bright Future.* New York: Broadway Books.

Cassel, C. K. 2000. "In Defense of a Department of Geriatrics." *Annals of Internal Medicine* 133:297–301.

———. 2005. *Medicare Matters: What Geriatric Medicine Can Teach American Health Care.* Berkeley: University of California Press.

———. 2010. "Robert Butler's Legacy." *Health Affairs Blog.* August 30.

Cassel, C. K., H. J. Cohen, E. B. Larson, R. M. Leipzig, and D. E. Meier, eds. 2003. *Geriatric Medicine: An Evidence-Based Approach.* New York: Springer-Verlag, 2003.

Castle Connelly Medical Ltd. "Best Doctors." http://www.castleconnelly.com/doctors/full.cfin?

Center to Advance Palliative Care. "Diane E. Meier, MD, FACP." http://www.capc.org/about-capc.

Christ, A. E. 1961. "Attitudes Toward Death Among a Group of Acute Geriatric Psychiatric Patients." *Journal of Gerontology* 16:56–59.

"Christine K. Cassel." n.d. *World Health Professions Alliance.* http://www.whpa.org/whpcr2010/bio_Christine_Cassel.htm.

Christy, N. P. 1995. "Virginia Kneeland Frantz 1896–1967." *P&S Journal* 15 (2).

Clarfield, A. M. 2009. "Review." *Journal of the American Medical Association* 301 (January 7): 107–8.

Cohen, R. A. 1963. Preface. In *Human Aging: A Biological and Behavioral Study.* Edited by J. E. Birren, R. N. Butler, S. W. Greenhouse, L. Sokoloff, and M. R. Yarrow, ix–x. Bethesda, Md.: National Institute of Mental Health.

Cole, J. O., and R. W. Gerard. 1959. *Psychopharmacology: Problems in Evaluation.* Washington, D.C.: National Academy of Sciences-National Research Council.

Cole, J. R. 2010 *The Great American University: Its Rise to Preeminence, Its Indispensable National Role, Why It Must Be Protected.* New York: Public Affairs.

Cole, J. R., E. G. Barber, and S. R. Graubard, eds. 1994. *The Research University in a Time of Discontent.* Baltimore: Johns Hopkins University Press.

Cole, J. R., and J. A. Lipton, J. A. 1977. "The Reputation of American Medical Schools." *Social Forces* 55:662–84.

Cole, T. R., and S. Gadow. 1987. *What Does It Mean to Grow Old? Reflections from the Humanities.* Durham: Duke University Press.

Cole, T. R., and M. G. Winkler, eds. 1994. *Oxford Book of Aging.* New York: Oxford University Press.

Coles, R. 1967. "The Jamesian Psychoanalyst." *Contemporary Psychoanalysis* 3:167–71.

A College Program in Action: A Review of Working Principles at Columbia College. 1946. New York: Columbia University Press.

Columbia University. n.d. "The Core Curriculum: History of the Core." http://www.college.columbia.edu/core/timeline.

Cooper, R. A. 2008. *OECD Health Working Paper No. 37. The U.S. Physician Workforce: Where Do We Stand?* Paris: OECD.

Cournand, A. 1989. "Dickinson Woodruff Richards: October 30, 1895–February 23, 1973." In *Biographical Memoirs.* Vol. 58. Washington, D.C.: National Academy of Sciences.

Cowdry, E. V., ed. 1939. *The Problems of Ageing: Biological and Medical Aspects.* Baltimore: Williams & Wilkins.

Cross, T. C. 1995. *An Oasis of Order: The Core Curriculum at Columbia College.* New York: Office of the Dean, Columbia College.

"D. M. Bullard Jr., 66, Led Psychiatric Unit." 1995. *New York Times.* August 12. http://www.nytimes.com/1995/08/12/obituaries/dm-bullard-jr-66-led-psychiatric-unit.html.

Damrosch, D. S. 1966. "Citation and presentation of the Academy Medal to Rustin McIntosh, M.D." *Bulletin of the New York Academy of Medicine* 42 (10): 935–36.

"Decline of Baby Boomers in America." n.d. *Internet Learning Center.* http://www.ilcusa.org/pages/projects/age-boom.php/.

DeGroot, L. J., ed. 1966. *Medical Care: Social and Organizational Aspects.* Springfield, Ill.: C. C. Thomas.

Dewey, J. 1916. *Democracy and Education: An Introduction to the Philosophy of Education.* New York: Macmillan.

Disch, R., ed. 1988. *Twenty-Five Years of the Life Review: Theoretical and Practical Considerations.* New York: Haworth Press.

Dobrof, R. 1984. "Introduction: A Time for Reclaiming the Past." In *The Uses of Reminiscence.* Edited by M. Kaminsky. New York: Haworth Press.

"Dr. Robert Butler, First NIA Director, Strayed from Original Goal." n.d. *Immor-Talist Manifesto.* http://immortalism.com/.

Doering, William V. E. 1990–91. Interview with James J. Bohning. "William Von Eggers Doering." 0085, Philadelphia and Cambridge. November and May. Chemical Heritage Foundation.

"Does Barbara Walters Have a Boyfriend?" n.d. *ChaChaAnswers.* http://www.chacha.com/question/does-barabara-walters-have-a-boyfriend.

Doron, I., and I. Apter. 2010. "The Debate Around the Need for an International Convention on the Rights of Older Persons. *Gerontologist* 50:586–93.

Downs, H. 1983. "Foreword." In *Aging & Mental Health: Consumer's Edition.* By R. N. Butler and M. I. Lewis. New York: New American Library.

Dreifus, C. 2006. "A Conversation with Robert N. Butler." *New York Times.* November 14.

Dupree, A. H. 1986. *Science in the Federal Government: A History of Policies and Activities.* 2d ed. Baltimore: John Hopkins University Press.

"Education: Columbia in the Heat." 1943. *Time Magazine.* July 19. http//www.time.com/time/magazine/article/0,9171,777876,00.html.

Elder, G. H. 1974. *Children of the Great Depression: Social Change in Life Experience.* Chicago: University of Chicago Press.

———. 1999. "The Life Course and Aging: Some Reflections." Distinguished Scholar Lecture prepared for the aging section of the American Sociological Association, August 10.

Elinson, J., E. Padilla, and M. E. Perkins. 1967. *Public Image of Mental Health Services.* New York: Mental Health Materials Center.

Elphick, P. 2006. *Liberty: The Ships That Won the War.* Washington, D.C.: Naval Institute Press.

"Episcopal Bishop Paul Moore Jr., 83, Dies; Strong Voice on Social and Political Issues." 2003. *New York Times,* May 2.

Ernst, F. H., W. A. Oliver, A. Simon, and N. Malamud. 1956. "Geriatric Patients in a Mental Hospital." *California Medicine* 84:172–75.

Fairhurst, G. T., and R. A. Sarr. 2006. *The Art of Framing*. San Francisco: Jossey-Bass.

Fallows, J. 2011. "Learning to Love the (Shallow, Divisive, Unreliable) News Media." *Atlantic* 307:36, 41.

Farber, L. H. 1966. *The Ways of the Will: Essays Toward a Psychology and Psychopathology of Will*. New York: Basic Books.

Fein, E. 1994. "Gaps in Geriatric Medicine Alarm Health Professionals." *New York Times*. May 16. http://www.nytimes.com/1994/05/16/us/gaps-in-geriatric-medicine-alarm-health-professionals.html.

———. 1995. "Dr. Thomas C. Chalmers, a President of Mt. Sinai, Dies at 78." *New York Times*. December 29. http://www.nytimes.com/1995/12/29/nyregion/dr-thomas-c-chalmers-a-president-of-mt-sinai-dies-at-78.html.

Fein, R., and G. I. Weber. 1971. *Financing Medical Education*. New York: McGraw-Hill.

Felknor, B. L., ed. 1999. *The U.S. Merchant Marine at War: 1775–1945*. Annapolis: U.S. Naval Institute Press.

Fernandez-Ballesteros, R., et al. 2011. "Productivity in Old Age." *Research in Aging* 33:205–26.

Fillit, H., and R. N. Butler. 2009. "The Frailty Identity Crisis." *Journal of the American Geriatrics Society* 57:348–52.

Finch, C. E. 1994. *Longevity, Senescence and the Genome*. Chicago: University of Chicago Press.

———. 2009. "Review of *Longevity Revolution*." *Gerontologist* 49:577–79.

Fiske, M. 1960. *Some Social Dimensions of Psychiatric Disorders in Old Age*. San Francisco: Langley Porter Neuropsychiatric Institute.

Flexner, A. 1910. *Medical Education in the United States and Canada: A Report to the Carnegie Foundation for the Advancement of Teaching*. Bulletin 4. Boston: Merrymount Press.

Fornal, S. L. 2011. "Our Uncivil Discourse." *Ellenville Journal*. http://www.ellenvillejournal.com/2011/02/03/nws/1102038.html.

Fox, P. J. 1989. "From Senility to Alzheimer's Disease: The Rise of the Alzheimer's Disease Movement." *Milbank Quarterly* 67:58–102.

FrameWorks Institute. 2002. *Framing Public Issues*. Washington, D.C.

Frazier, L. D., K. Hooker, and I. C. Siegler. 1993. "Longitudinal Studies of Aging in Social and Psychological Gerontology." *Reviews in Clinical Gerontology* 3:415–26.

Freedman, M. 2006–07. "The Social-Purpose Career: Baby Boomers, Civic Engagement, and the Next Stage of Work." *Generations* 30:43–46.

Freund, K. 2010. "The Loss of Robert Butler." http://newsletter.itnamerica.org/ITNAmerica/EnRoute/EnRouteJuly2010.html#Butler.

Friedan, B. 1985. "The Mystique of Age." In *Productive Aging: Enhancing Vitality in Later Life*. Edited by R. N. Butler and H. P. Gleason. New York: Springer.

———. 1993. *The Fountain of Age*. New York: Simon and Schuster.

Fries, J. F. 1983. "Compression of Morbidity." *Milbank Memorial Fund Quarterly* 61:397–419.

Galenson, D. W. 2006. *Old Masters and Young Geniuses: The Two Life Cycles of Artistic Creativity*. Princeton: Princeton University Press.

Gavrilov, L., and N. Gavrilova. 2008. "Review of *The Longevity Revolution*." *New England Journal of Medicine* 358:2187–88.

George, C. 2010. "Houston Centenarians Celebrate, and Reflect on 100 Years." *Houston Chronicle*. June 17.

Gilleard, C., and P. Higgs. 2010. "Frailty, Disability, and Old Age." *Health* 15:475–490.

———. 2011. "Ageing Abjection and Embodiment in the Fourth Age." *Journal of Aging Studies* 25:135–42.

Gilman, S., and N. L. Foster. 1996. "The Alzheimerization of Aging: A Response." *Gerontologist* 36:9–10.

Ginzberg, E. 1985. *American Medicine: The Power Shift*. Totowa, N.J.: Rowman & Allanheld.

———. 2000. *Teaching Hospitals and the Urban Poor*. New Haven: Yale University Press.

Ginzberg, E., H. W. Berliner, and M. Ostow. 1993. *Changing U.S. Health Care*. Boulder: Westview Press

Ginzberg, E., and A. B. Dutka. 1989. *The Financing of Biomedical Research*. Baltimore: Johns Hopkins University Press.

Giroux, H. A. 2011. "Public Intellectuals, the Politics of Clarity, and the Crisis of Language." *State of Nature: An Online Journal of Radical Ideas*. http://www .stateofnature.org/publicIntellectualsThePolitics.html.

Gitlin, T. 1993. *The Sixties: Years of Hope, Days of Rage*. New York: Bantam,

Glaser, H. H., M. C. Heagarty, D. M. Bullard, and E. C. Pivchik. 1968. "Physical and Psychological Development of Children with Early Failure to Thrive." *Journal of Pediatrics* 73:690–98.

Glaser, V. 2003. "Organizational Profile: International Longevity Center. *Journal of Anti-Aging Medicine* 6:117–20.

Goodman, E. 2011. "Now Is the Time to Redefine Aging." *Wilmington (Ohio) News Journal*, January 5. http://www.wnewsj.com/main/asp?SectionID=42& SubSectionD=201&ArticleID:18773.

Gordon, L. 2009. *Dorothea Lange: A Life Beyond Limits*. New York: Norton.

Gostin, L. O. 2010. "The Unconscionable Health Gap: A Global Plan for Justice." *Lancet* 375:1504–5.

Gower, P. L., ed. 2005. *New Research on the Psychology of Fear.* New York: Nova Science Publishers.

Graham, H. D., and N. Diamond. 1997. *The Rise of American Research Universities.* Baltimore: Johns Hopkins University Press.

Grant, B. 2011. "The Ghost of Personalized Medicine." *The Scientist.* http://the-scientist.com/2011/06/14/the-ghost-of-personalized-medicine.

Greenberg, R. M., and O. T. Fein. 1999. "Dr. David E. Rogers and His Legacy." *Journal of Urban Health* 76:10–17.

Grob, G. N. 1987. "The Forging of Mental Health Policy in America: World War II to New Frontier." *Journal of the History of Medicine and Allied Sciences* 42:410–46.

Group for the Advancement of Psychiatry (GAP). 1950. *The Social Responsibility of Psychiatry: A Statement of Orientation.* New York: Group for the Advancement of Psychiatry.

——. 1954. *Considerations Regarding the Loyalty Oath as a Manifestation of Current Social Tension and Anxiety.* New York: Group for the Advancement of Psychiatry.

——. 1955. *Report on Homosexuality with Particular Emphasis on This Problem in Governmental Agencies.* New York: Group for the Advancement of Psychiatry.

——. 1957. *Psychiatric Aspects of School Desegregation.* New York: Group for the Advancement of Psychiatry.

Gruenberg, E. M. 1977. "The Failures of Success." *Milbank Memorial Fund Quarterly/Health and Society* 55:3–24.

Gruman, G. 1978. "Cultural Origins of Present-Day Ageism." In *Aging and the Elderly.* Edited by S. F. Spicker, K. M. Woodward, and D. D. Van Tassel. Atlantic Highlands, N.J.: Humanities Press.

Gutierrez-Lobos, K., M. Scherer, and P. Anderer. 2002. "The Influence of Age on the Female/Male Ratio of Treated Incidence Rates in Depression." *BCM Psychiatry* 2:3.

Haak, J. L., and K. Kaye. 2009. "Personal Psychotherapy During Residency Training: A Survey of Psychiatric Residents." *Academic Psychiatry* 33:323–26.

Haber, C. 2004. "Life Extension and History." *Journals of Gerontology: Biological Science* 59:B515–22.

Haight, B. K., and B. S. Haight. 2007. *The Handbook of Structured Life Review.* Baltimore: Health Professions Press.

Hahn, T. 2005, November 19. "Myrna Lewis Wrote Books About Sexuality and Aging." *Star Tribune.* http://www.startribune.com/templates/Print_This_Story?sid=11596966.

Hanisch, Carol. 1970. "The Personal Is Political." In *Notes from the Second Year: Women's Liberation*. New York: Sulasmith Firestone & Anne Koeht.

Hannaway, C. 2008. *Biomedicine in the Twentieth Century: Practices, Policies, and Politics*. Amsterdam: IOS Press.

Harden, V. A. 1986. *Inventing NIH: Federal Biomedical Research Policy, 1887–1937*. Baltimore: Johns Hopkins University Press.

Hareven, T. K. 1994. "Aging and Generational Relations: A Historical and Life Course Perspective." *Annual Review of Sociology* 20:437–61.

Hartocollis, A. 2010. "Getting Into Med School Without Hard Sciences." *New York Times*. July 29.

Hatch, L. R. 2000. *Beyond Gender Differences: Adaptation to Aging in Life Course Perspective*. Amityville, N.Y.: Baywood Publishing.

Hausman, K. 2004. "Pioneering Psychiatrist, Psychoanalyst Judd Marmor Dies at Age 93." *Psychiatric News* 39:2.

Hayflick, L., and H. R. Moody. 2003. *Has Anyone Ever Died of Old Age?* New York: International Longevity Center.

Hayflick, L., and P. Moorhead. 1961. "The Serial Cultivation of Human Diploid Cell Strains." *Experimental Cell Research* 25:585–621.

Hazzard, W. R. 1979. "An American's Ode to British Geriatrics." *Age and Ageing* 8:141–43.

———. 2000. "The Department of Internal Medicine: Hub of the Academic Health Center Response to the Aging Imperative." *Annals of Internal Medicine* 133:293–96.

———. 2004. "Capturing the Power of Academic Medicine to Enhance Health and Health Care of the Elderly in the USA." *Geriatrics and Gerontology International* 4:5–14.

Healy, D. 2004. *The Creation of Psychopharmacology*. Cambridge: Harvard University Press.

"The Heinz Awards: Julius Richmond Profile." 2008. http://www.heinzawards.net/recipients/julius-richmond

"The Heinz Awards: Robert Butler Profile." 2003. http://www.heinzawards.net/recipients/robert-butler.

Henry, C. P. 1999. *Ralph Bunche: Model Negro or American Other?* New York: New York University, Press.

"Henry Lewis Gates, Jr." 2011. http://prelectur.stanford.edu/lecturers/gates.

Hevesi, D. 2007. "Marian Radke-Yarrow, Child Psychology Researcher, Dies at 89." *New York Times*, May 23. http://www.nytimes.com/2007/05/23/health/23yarrow.html.

———. 2008. "Paul G. Rogers, 'Mr. Health' in Congress, Is Dead at 87." *New York Times*. October 15. http://www.nytimes.com/2008/10/15/us/15rogers.html.

Heyssel, R. M., J. R. Gaintner, I. W. Kues, A. A. Jones, and S. H. Lipstein. 1984. "Decentralized Management in a Teaching Hospital." *New England Journal of Medicine* 310:1477–80.

Hine, C., L. Margolis, A. Simon, A. Shick, and N. T. Burbridge. 1952. "Effects of Alcohol in Small Doses and Tetraethylthiuramdisuphide (Antabus) on the Cerebral Blood Flow and Cerebral Metabolism." *Journal of Pharmacological Experimental Therapy*, 253–60.

Hirsch, E. D., J. F. Kett, and J. S. Trefil. 2002. *The New Dictionary of Cultural Literacy*. 3d ed. Boston: Houghton Mifflin.

"History: Making a Difference for Older Americans: 1950–Today." n.d. National Council on the Aging. http://www.ncoa.org/about-ncoa/ncoa-history.html.

Hodgson, G. 2000. *The Gentleman from New York: Daniel Patrick Moynihan—a Biography*. Boston: Houghton Mifflin Harcourt.

Hofstadter, R. 1963. *Anti-Intellectualism in American Life*. New York: Vintage.

Holzman, P. S. 2000. "Seymour S. Kety and the Genetics of Schizophrenia." *Neuropsychopharmacology* 25. http://www.nature.com/npp/journal/v25/n3/full/1395719a.html.

"Howard Fillit MD: Executive Profile & Biography—Business Week." *Business Week*. http://investing.businessweek.com/research/stocks/private/person.asp?personId=665894&privcapId=2101814&previousCapId=2101814&previousTitle=Institute%20for%20the%20Study%20of%20Aging,%20The.

Hughes, T. P., and A. C. Hughes. 1990. *Lewis Mumford: Public Intellectual*. New York: Oxford University Press.

Hyland, L. M. 2010. "Celebrating Dr. Butler: ILC's Founder Dies at 83." *INPEA web*. http://www.inpea.net/images/RobertButler_ILC_Tribute.pdf.

Ignatieff, M. 1997. "The Decline and Fall of the Public Intellectual." *Queen's Quarterly* 104:395–403.

Ihara, K. ca. 1998. *Japan's Policies on Long-term Care for the Aged: The Gold Plan and the Long-term Care Insurance Plan*. New York: International Longevity Center.

Institute of Medicine. 1996. *Primary Care*. Washington, D.C.: National Academy Press.

———. 2008. *Retooling for an Aging America: Building the Health Care Workforce*. Washington, D.C.: National Academies Press.

International Longevity Center (ILC). 1999. *The Aging Factor in Health and Disease*. New York: ILC-USA.

———. 2000. *Biomarkers of Aging: From Primitive Organisms to Man*. New York: ILC.

————. 2002. *Clinical Trials and Older Persons: The Need for Greater Representation.* New York: ILC.

————. 2003. *Unjust Desserts: Financial Realities of Older Women.* New York: ILC.

————. 2011. "ILC-USA Gains Greater Independence." http://www.zorgvoolater.com/ip/uploads/tblvsiedocumenten/ILC U...

————. n.d. "Board of Directors." http://www.ilcusa.org/pages/about-us/board-of-directors.php.

————. n.d. "Staff and Associates." http://www.ilcusa.org/pages/about-us/staff-associates.php.

International Longevity Center Global Alliance. 2009. *Global Aging Report.* http://www.ilcjapan.org/alliance/doc/Global_Aging_Report_090212.pdf.

"Internationally Known Urologist James Glenn Dies." 2009. http://www.kentucky.com/2009/06/11/826500.

"Interview with C. Everett Koop, M.D., the U.S. Surgeon General." 1982. *Hospital Progress,* 20–21.

Isbell, L. A. 2009. *The Fruit, the Tree, and the Serpent.* Cambridge: Harvard University Press.

"Jack Ossofsky, 66; Led Council on Aging" 1992. *New York Times.* September 6. http://www.nytimes.com/1992/09/06/obituaries/jack-ossofsky-66-led-council-on-aging.html.

"Jack Weinberg, M.D., 1910–1982." 1983. *American Journal of Psychiatry* 140:1239–40.

Jackson, H. C. 1971. "National Caucus on the Black Aged: A Progress Report." *International Journal of Aging and Human Development* 2:226–31.

Jackson, K. T., ed. 1995. *The Encyclopedia of New York City.* New Haven: Yale University Press.

Jacoby, R. 1987. *The Last Intellectuals.* New York: Noonday Press.

"Japan in the Year 2000: Preparing Japan for an Age of Internationalization, the Aging Society and Maturity." 1983. *Japan Times.*

John A. Hartford Foundation. 2005. "A Brief History of Geriatrics." http://www.jhartford.org/ar2005html/2_a_brief_ history.html.

"John W. Rowe '66, HON '02, MD." 2010. http://www.canisius.edu/campaign/rowe.asp.

"John W. Rowe." 2010. The Rockefeller Foundation. http://www.rockefellerfoundation.org/about-us/board-trustees/john-w-rowe/.

Johnson, M. L. 2011. Private communication.

Johnson, S. 1982. "Geriatrics Field Offers a Promising Future." *New York Times.* October 12.

Johnson, T. 2010. "'Dear Abby' Struggles with Alzheimer's." *ABCNews.com*. http:// abcnews.go.com/GMA/Dr.Johnson/story?id=12809&page=1.

Judd, P. H., and T. H. McGlashan. 2003. *A Developmental Model of Borderline Personality Disorder*. Washington, D.C.: American Psychiatric Publishing.

Kabaservice, G. 2004. *The Guardians: Kingman Brewster, His Circle, and the Rise of the Liberal Establishment*. New York: Henry Holt.

Kadushin, C. 1974. *The American Intellectual Elite*. Boston: Little, Brown.

Kaminsky, M. 1984a. "Transfiguring Life." In *Uses of Reminiscence: New Ways of Working with Older Adults*. Edited by M. Kaminsky, 3–14. New York: Haworth Press.

Kaminsky, M., ed. 1984b. *Uses of Reminiscence: New Ways of Working with Older Adults*. New York: Haworth Press.

"Karl M. Bowman, Psychiatrist, 84." 1973. *New York Times*. March 4.

Karlin, B. E., A. M. Zeiss, and J. F. Burris. 2010. "Providing Care to Older Americans in the Department of Veterans Affairs." *Generations* 34 (2): 6–8.

Kashatus, W. C. 2010. *Dapper Dan Flood: The Controversial Life of a Congressional Power Broker*. University Park: Pennsylvania State University Press.

Kastor, J. A. 2010. *The National Institutes of Health, 1991–2008*. New York: Oxford University Press.

Katzman, R. 1976. "The Prevalence and Malignancy of Alzheimer Disease: A Major Killer." *Archives of Neurology* 33:217–18.

Katzman, R., and K. L. Bick. 2000. *Alzheimer Disease: The Changing View*. San Diego: Academic Press.

Katzman, R., R. Terry, and K. Bick, eds. 1978. *Alzheimer's Disease: Senile Dementia and Related Disorders*. New York: Raven Press.

Keane, J. 2008. "Civil Society and Ageing." *Nova Acta Leopoldina* 99:1–10.

Kennedy, D. M. 1999. *Freedom from Fear: The American People in Depression and War, 1929–1945*. New York: Oxford University Press.

Kennedy, T. J. 1994. "James Augustine Shannon: August 9, 1904–May 20, 1994." *Biographical Memoirs*. Vol. 65. Washington, D.C.: National Academies Press.

Kenyon, G., E. Bohlmeijer, and W. L. Randall. 1995, *Storying Later Life: Issues, Investigations, and Interventions in Narrative Gerontology*. Oxford: Oxford University Press.

Kerschner, H., and J. A. Pegues. 1998. "Productive Aging: A Quality of Life Agenda." *Journal of the American Dietetic Association* 98:1445–48.

Kety, S. 1999. "Mental Illness and the Sciences of Brain and Behavior." *Nature Medicine* 5 (10): 1113–16.

"Khan, Princess Y. A." n.d. Women's International Center. http://www.wic.org/bio /pkhan.htm.

Kirk, R. 1982. "Promises and Perils of Christian Politics." *Intercollegiate Review* 18:13–23.

Kleyman, P. 2010. "Robert N. Butler, MD, 83, Dies." *Generations Beat Online.* July 7. http://network.newamericanmedia.org/gbo/archives/10_11.

———. 2011. "The Legacies of Memory: What Elders Bring to the Future—Butler Reviews Life Review." *American Society on Aging.* http://www.asaging.org/at /at-214/legacymem.html.

Kline, N. 1956. *Psychopharmacology.* Washington, D.C.: American Association for the Advancement of Science Publications.

Kohut, N. 2000. *Analysis of the Self: Systematic Approach to Treatment of Narcissistic Personality Disorders.* New York: International Universities Press.

Koop, C. E. 1983. "Toward a Philosophy of Aging for the Public Health Professions." *Public Health Reports* 98:203–6.

———. 1984. "Exploring the Myths and Realities of Aging and Health." *Aging* 3:5–9.

Kopin, I. J. 1995. Interview with Seymour Kety. December 12.

Kraemer, S. 2006. *Science and Technology Policy in the United States: Open Systems in Action.* New Brunswick, N.J.: Rutgers University Press.

Kunz, J. A., and F. G. Soltys. 2007. *Transformational Reminiscence: Life Story Work.* New York: Springer.

Lachin, J. M., and J. Greenhouse. n.d. "Samuel W. Greenhouse: 1918–2000." *Statisticians in History.* http://www.amstat.org/about/statisticiansinhistory/index .cfm?fuseaction=biosinfo&BioID=5.

Lakoff, G. 2004. *Don't Think of an Elephant! Know Your Values and Frame the Debate.* White River Junction, Vt.: Chelsea Green Publishing.

LaMarche, G. 2011a. "About Atlantic." http://www.atlanticphilanthropies.org /current/aboutatlantic.

———. 2011b. "The Billionaire Who Wasn't." http://www.atlanticphilanthropies .org/current/billionaire-who-wasn't.

Lambino, A. 2009. "Naming and Framing Policy Issues." http://blogs.worldbank .org/naming-and-framing-policy-issues.

Landrigan, P. J., B. Sonawane, R. N. Butler, L. Trasande, R. Callan, and D. Droller. 2005. "Early Environmental Origins of Neurodegenerative Disease in Later Life." *Environmental Health Perspectives* 113:1230–33.

Lasch, C. 1979. *The Culture of Narcissism.* New York: Norton.

Laslett, P. 1989. *A Fresh Map of Life.* London: Weidenfeld & Nicholson.

Laursen, E. 2010. "Robert Butler and the Battle for Social Security." Gray Panthers Collection, Temple University Libraries accession 835. http://peoplespension.info shop.org/blogs-mu/2010/07/07/robert-butler-and-the-battle-for-social-security/.

———. 2012. *The People's Pension: The Struggle to Defend Social Security Since Reagan.* Oakland: AK Press.

Lederberg, Joshua. n.d. "Research and the Culture of Incrementalism." *21st* C. http:www.columbia.edu/cu/21stC/issue-1.1/nobel.htm.

Lee, T. 2010. "Intrepid Exploring." *Journal of Aging, Humanities, and the Arts* (December): 18–29.

Lepore, J. 2011. "Twilight." *New Yorker* 208 (March 14): 30–35.

Leslie, R. 2004. "Anti-aging Medicine." *Journal of Gerontology: Biological Sciences* 59: B540–42.

Lesparre, M. 1976. "Interview with Robert N. Butler, M.D., Director, National Institute on Aging." *Journal of the American Hospital Association* 50:50.

Levine, J. 2004 *Do You Remember Me? A Father, a Daughter, and a Search for the Self.* New York: Simon and Schuster.

Lewis, D. L. 2000. *W. E. B. DuBois: The Fight for Equality and the American Century, 1919–1963.* New York: Holt.

Lewis, M. I. 2005. *A Proactive Approach to Women's Concerns: Women's Longevity Groups and Funds.* New York: International Longevity Center.

Lewis, M. I., and R. N. Butler. 1974. "Life-Review Therapy: Putting Memories to Work in Individual and Group Psychotherapy. *Geriatrics* 29:165–69, 172–73.

Lewis, S. 1925. *Arrowsmith.* New York: Harcourt, Brace.

Libow, L. S. 2004. "Geriatrics in the United States—Baby Boomers' Boon?" *New England Journal of Medicine* 352:750–52.

Lidz, T. 1968. *The Person: His Development Throughout the Life Cycle.* New York: Basic Books.

Liebig, P. S. 1983. "Mental Health Care of the Elderly in a Time of Scarcity." *Administration in Mental Health* 11:124–32.

Lim, E. T. 2008. *The Anti-Intellectual Presidency: The Decline of Presidential Rhetoric from George Washington to George W. Bush.* New York: Oxford University Press.

Lindenmeyer, K. 2005. *The Greatest Generation Grows Up: American Childhood in the 1930s.* Chicago: Ivan R. Dee.

Lippmann, W. 1922. *Public Opinion.* New York: Macmillan.

Lockett, B. 1983. *Aging, Politics, and Research: Setting the Federal Agenda for Research on Aging.* New York: Springer.

Loeb, R. F. 1963. "Reflections on Undergraduate Medical Education." *British Medical Journal* 2 (5357): 579–80.

Longman, P. 1987. *Born to Pay.* Boston: Houghton Mifflin.

Lowenthal, M. F. 1964a. *Lives in Distress.* New York: Basic Books.

———. 1964b. "Social Isolation and Mental Illness in Old Age." *American Socio-logical Review* 29:54–70.

Ludmerer, K. M. 1999. *Time to Heal: American Medical Education from the Turn of the Center to the Era of Managed Care.* New York: Oxford University Press.

Luijendijk, H. J., J. F. van den Berg, M. J. Dekker, H. R. van Tuikl, W. Otte, F. Smit, and H. Tiemeier. 2008. "Incidence and Recurrence of Late-Life Depression." *Archives of General Psychiatry* 65:1394–1401.

Macklin, E. A., A. Simon, and G. H. Crook. 1953 "Psychotic Reactions in Problem Drinkers Treated with Disulfiram (Antabuse)." *Archives of Neurology and Psychiatry* 69:415–26.

Macnicol, J. 2006. *Age Discrimination.* Cambridge: Cambridge University Press.

Maddox, G. L. 1968. "Persistence of Life Style Among the Elderly." In *Middle Age and Aging.* Edited by B. L. Neugarten. Chicago: University of Chicago Press.

Magee, M. 2010. *Healthy Commentary* blog. http://healthcommentary.org?page_id=3035.

Mahler, M., F. Pine, and A. Bergman, A. 1975. *The Psychological Birth of the Infant: Symbiosis and Individuation.* New York: Basic Books.

Marcello, P. C. 2004. *Ralph Nader: A Biography.* Westport: Greenwood Press.

Margolis, L. H. 1957. "Pharmacotherapy in Psychiatry: A Review." *Annals of the New York Academy of Sciences* 66:698–718.

Margolis, L. H., R. N. Butler, and A. Fischer. 1955. "Nonrecurring Chlorpromazine Dermatitis." *AMA Archives of Dermatology* 72:72–73.

Marmot, M. 2006. *Why Care? How Status Affects Our Health and Longevity.* Harold Hatch Lecture in Geriatrics and Gerontology. New York: International Longevity Center and Brookdale Department of Geriatrics and Adult Development of Mount Sinai School of Medicine.

Martin, J. 2002. *Nader: Crusader, Spoiler, Icon.* New York: Basic Books.

Martineau, K. 2009. "Dr. Robert Butler '49 Advocates for Older People." *Columbia College Today: Alumni Profiles.* http://www.college.columbia.edu/cct/jan_feb09/alumni_profileso.

Matusow, A. J. 1985. *The Unraveling of America: A History of Liberalism in the 1960s.* New York: Perennial.

Mayer, C. 2010. "Robert Butler, Guru of Growing Old." *Time Magazine.* July 7. http://www.time.com/time/magazine/article/0,9171,2002533,00.html.

McCaughey, R. A. 2003 *Stand, Columbia.* New York: Columbia University Press.

———. 2004. "Columbia in the 'American Century.'" *Timelines 1945–1964.* http://beatl.barnard.columbia.edu/stand_columbia/Timeline1946–64.html.

McDavid, T. 2010. *Blog for Causes.* http://blog/causescalendar.com/?p=121.

McDermott, W. 1980. "Medicine: The Public Good and One's Own." *World Health Forum* 1:124.

McElvaine, R. 1993. *The Great Depression, 1929–1941*. New York: Times Books.

———, ed. 2008. *Down and Out in the Great Depression: Letters from the Forgotten Man*. Chapel Hill: University of North Carolina Press.

McGlashan, T. H., and W. S. Fenton. 1998. "Frieda Fromm-Reichmann, 1889–1957." *American Journal of Psychiatry* 155:123.

McGovern, J. R. 2001. *And a Time for Hope: Americans in the Great Depression*. Westport, Conn.: Praeger.

McHugh, William. 1969. "Interview with Bertram S. Brown." Oral History Interview—JFK#2, 1/29/1969, 13.

McNeill, W. H. 1991. *Hutchins' University: A Memoir of the University of Chicago, 1929–1950*. Chicago: University of Chicago Press.

Mellan, O. 2010. "Longevity, Your Clients, and You." *Investment Advisor* (June): 7–8.

Menninger, W. C. 1948. "Notices and Bulletins: Group for the Advancement of Psychiatry." *Psychosomatic Medicine* 10 (1): 54–56.

Mensh, I. 1974. "Ageism." *PsycCRITIQUES* 19:405.

Merrick, E. L., C. M. Horgan, D. Hodgkin, D. W. Garnick, S. F. Houghton, and L. Panas. 2008. "Unhealthy Drinking Patterns in Older Adults: Prevalence and Associated Characteristics." *Journal of the American Geriatrics Society* 58:214–23.

Metchnikoff, E. 1903. *The Nature of Man*. New York: Putnam.

Meyer, E. L. 2007. "Hurricane Steve Moves On." *Columbia College Today*. http://www.college.columbia/edu/cct_archive/jul_aug07/features1.php.

Michael, J. 2000. *Anxious Intellects: Academic Professionals, Public Intellectuals, and Enlightenment Values*. Durham: Duke University Press.

Miller, R. A. 2001. "Biomarkers of Aging." *Science: Science of Aging Knowledge Environment* 1: pe2.

———. 2002. "Extending Life: Scientific Prospects and Political Obstacles." *Milbank Quarterly* 80:163–64.

Mills, C. W. 1959. *The Sociological Imagination*. New York: Oxford University Press.

Minnesota Psychiatric Society. n.d. "Detailed History of Mental Health." http://www.mnpsychosoc.org/history%20appendix.pdf.

"Mission & History." n.d. 92d Street Y, New York. http://www.92y.org/content/about_the_y_mission_history.asp.

Moen, P., D. Dempster-McClain, and R. M. Williams. 1992. "Successful Aging: A Life-Course Perspective on Women's Multiple Roles and Health." *American Journal of Sociology* 97:1612–38.

Moody, H. R. 1988. "Twenty-five Years of the Life Review: Where Did We Come From? Where Are We Going?" *Journal of Gerontological Social Work* 12 (3–4): 7–21.

Moody, H. R., and W. A. Achenbaum. Forthcoming. *Leaving a Legacy*.

Morrow, A. 2009. "The Five Stages of Life Review: Preparing for Death with Life Review." http://dying.about.com/od/thedyingprocess/a/life_review.htm.

Morrow-Howell, N., J. Hinterlong, and M. Sherraden, eds. 2001. *Productive Aging: Concepts and Challenges*. Baltimore: Johns Hopkins University Press.

Mount Sinai Medical Center. Martha Stewart Center for Living. n.d. http://www .mountsinai.org/patient-care/services-areas/geriatrics-and-aging/areas-of-care/ martha-stewart-center-for-living.

"Mount Sinai School of Medicine: History." n.d. http://www.mssm.edu/about-us /who-we-are/history.

Mushkin, S. J. 1979. *Biomedical Research: Costs and Benefits*. Cambridge, Mass.: Ballinger.

Nannes, C. H. 1957. *The National Presbyterian Church & Center*. Baltimore: Vinmar Lithographing Company.

Nascher, I. L. 1914. *Geriatrics: The Diseases of Old Age and Their Treatment, Including Physiological Old Age, Home and Institutional Care, and Medico-Legal Relations*. Philadelphia: P. Blakiston & Sons.

National Cancer Act of 1971 (PL 92-218, December 23). 1971. "Findings and Declaration of Purpose," Section 404, a, 1. http://legislative.cancer.gov/history /phsa/1971.

National Institute on Aging (NIA). 1977. *Profiles of International Institutes with Programs in the Field of Aging*. Washington, D.C.: Government Printing Office.

———. 1978. With the advice of the National Advisory Council on Aging. *Our Future Selves: A Research Plan Toward Understanding Aging*. DHEW Publication 77-1096. Bethesda: Public Health Service.

———. 1980. "Senility Reconsidered: Treatment Possibilities for Mental Impairment in the Elderly." Task Force Special Communication. *Journal of the American Medical Association* 244:259–63.

———. 1982. *Toward an Independent Old Age: A National Plan for Research on Aging*. Washington, D.C.: Government Printing Office.

———. n.d. "Baltimore Longitudinal Study of Aging-Time Line." http://grc.nia .nih.gov/branches/blsa/butler.htm.

National Institutes of Health (NIH). 2010. "Important Events in NIMH History." *NIH Almanac*. http:www.nih.gov/about/almanac/organization/NIMH.htm.

National Library of Medicine. n.d. *The Donald S. Fredrickson Papers*. http:// profiles.nlm.nih.gov/ps/retrieve/Narrative/FF/p-nid/230.

National Research Council, Commission on Human Resources. 1976. *The 1976 Report of the Commission on a Study of National Needs for Biomedical and Behavioral Research Personnel*. Washington, D.C.: National Academy of Sciences.

Nelson, Bob. 1999. "Charles Dawson, Columbia Chemist Known for Work on Poison Ivy, 88." *Columbia University News*. http://columbia.edu/cu/pr/99/19536.htm.

Nelson, T. D., ed. 2002. *Ageism: Stereotyping and Prejudice Against Older Persons*. Cambridge: MIT Press.

Neugarten, B. L., ed. 1968. *Middle Age and Aging: A Reader in Social Psychology*. Chicago: University of Chicago Press.

———. 1974. "Age Groups in American Society and the Rise of the Young-Old." *Annals of the American Academy of Political and Social Sciences* 320 (September): 187–98.

Newton, D. 2010. "Ten Minutes with Robert Butler, MD." http://www.agingwellconsortium.com/writers-circle.html.

Nordhaus, W. D. 2002. *The Health of Nations: The Contribution of Improved Health to Living Standards*. Working Paper 8818. Cambridge, Mass.: National Bureau of Economic Research.

Norman, M. 1997. "The Man Who Saw Old Anew." *New York Times Magazine*. March 9. http://www.nytimes.com/1997/03/09/magazine/the-man-who-saw-old-anew.html.

Normile, D. 2004. "Older Scientists Win Majority of Funding." *Science* 303:1746.

Nuland, S. B. 2003. *Lost in America: A Journey with My Father*. New York: Knopf.

OBrien-Suric, N. 2010. "Honoring Bob Butler." *John A. Hartford Agenda*. http://www.jhartfound.org/blog/honoring-bob-butler/.

O'Connor, S. D., S. Prusiner, and K. Dychtwald. 2010. "The Age of Alzheimer's." *New York Times*. October 27. http://www.nytimes.com/2010/10/28/opinion/28oconnor.html.

Olshansky, S. J. 2009. "Aging in America in the Twenty-first Century. *Milbank Quarterly* 87:842–62.

Olshansky, S. J., B. A. Carnes, and R. N. Butler. 2003. "If Humans Were Built to Last." *Scientific American* 13 (2): 94–100.

Olshansky, S. J., D. J. Passaro, R. C. Hershow, J. Layden, B. A. Carnes, J. Brody, and D. S. Ludwig. 2005. "A Potential Decline in Life Expectancy in the United States in the 21st Century." *New England Journal of Medicine* 352:1138–45.

Olshansky, S. J., D. Perry, R. A. Miller, and R. N. Butler. 2006. "In Pursuit of the Longevity Dividend." *Scientist* 20:28–36.

O'Neill, W. (1974) 2005. *Coming Apart: An Informal History of the 1960s*. Chicago: Ivan Dee.

Oshinsky, D. M. 2005. *Polio: An American Story.* New York: Oxford University Press.

Osler, W. 1889. "Aequanimitas: Valedictory Address." Speech presented at the University of Pennsylvania, Philadelphia. May.

Ozarin, L. D. 1999. "William A. White, M.D.: A Distinguished Achiever." *Psychiatric News.* http://www.psychiatricnews.org/pnews/99–01–01/hx.html.

Padilla, E., J. Elinson, and M. E. Perkins. 1966. "Public Image of Mental Health Services." *American Journal of Public Health Nations Health* 56 (9): 1524–29.

Palladino, L. 2010. "Obituaries: Dr. Robert N. Butler '49, '53 P&S, Gerontologist and Author." *Columbia College Today.* September/October. http://www.college.columbia.edu/cct/sep_oct10/obituaries1.

Pan, C. X., E. Chai, and J. Farber. 2007. *Myths of the High Medical Cost of Old Age and Dying.* ILC-USA Report.

Paris, B. 2010. Remarks, Butler memorial service, All Saints' Unitarian Church, New York, N.Y., September 29.

Parker, R. 2005. *John Kenneth Galbraith: His Life, His Politics, His Economics.* Chicago: University of Chicago Press.

Parsons, T., and G. M. Platt. 1973. *The American University.* Cambridge: Harvard University Press.

Patterson, T. L., and D. V. Jeste. 1999. "The Potential Impact of the Baby-Boom Generation on Substance Abuse Among Elderly Persons." *Psychiatric Services* 50:184–88.

Pearce, J. 2005. "Virginia Apgar (1909–1974): Neurological Evaluation of the Newborn Infant." *European Neurology* 54 (3): 132–34.

———. 2007. "R. S. Paffenbarger, Jr., 84, Epidemiologist, Dies." *New York Times.* July 14. http://www.nytimes.com/2007/07/14/us/14paffenbarger.html.

Peck, R. L. 1996. " 'A Rough Old Age . . . '—Interview with Geriatrics Expert Robert N. Butler." *Nursing Homes: Long Term Management Care.* http://findarticles.com/p/articles/mi_m3830/is_n2/v45/ai_18113156/.

"People: R. Langley Porter: 1870–1965." 2010. http://history.library.ucsf.edu/porter.html.

Perlstein, S. 1988. "Transformation: Life Review and Communal Theatre." *Twenty-five Years of the Life Review: Theoretical and Practical Considerations.* New York: Haworth Press.

Perrott, G. St. J. 1946. "Selective Service Statistics and Some of Their Implications." *American Journal of Public Health* 36:339–46.

Perry, D. n.d. Interview by K. Jensen. [Audio tape recording]. "Longevity Science: Interview with Daniel Perry." http://www.sagecrossroads.net/files/EvolutionDan.pdf.

Peterson, P. G. 1988. *On Borrowed Time.* San Francisco: ICS Press.

———. 1999. *Gray Dawn.* New York: Times Books.

———. 2010. "Tax Aversion Syndrome and Our Deficit Future." *Wall Street Journal.* July 7.

Pifer, A., and D. L. Bronte. 1986. *Our Aging Society.* New York: Norton.

Poitier, S. 2000. *The Measure of a Man.* San Francisco: Harper.

Pollen, D. A. 1996. *Hannah's Heirs.* New York: Oxford University Press.

Portal of Geriatric Online Education. n.d. *POGOe Resources.* http://www.pogoe .org/node/453.

Posner, R. A. 2001. *Public Intellectuals: A Study of Decline.* Cambridge: Harvard University Press.

Post, S. G., and R. H. Binstock, eds. 2004. *The Fountain of Youth.* New York: Oxford University Press.

Potter, D. M. 1954. *People of Plenty: Economic Abundance and the American Character.* Chicago: University of Chicago Press.

Pratt, H. L. 1967. *The Gray Lobby.* Chicago: University of Chicago Press.

"The Prominence of Truth in the Priesthood." 2007. http://www.jknirp/com/prom inen.htm.

Proscio, T. 2010. *Winding Down the Atlantic Philanthropies.* Durham: Duke University, Sanford School of Public Policy.

"Prof./Dr. Anna Aslan, Bio and GEROVITAL Treatment." n.d. http://cosmetiques gerovital.com/aslaneng.html.

Rait, G., et al. 2009. "Recent Trends in the Incidence of Recorded Depression in Primary Care." *British Journal of Psychiatry* 195:520–24.

Randall, W. L., and A. E. McKim. 2008. *Reading Our Lives: The Poetics of Growing Old.* New York: Oxford University Press.

Redlener, I. 2009. *Americans at Risk.* New York: Random House.

"Remembering Reverend Peter Gomes, Beloved Harvard Spiritual Leader." 2011. http://www.thecrimsoncom/article/2011/3/2/gomes-harvard-university-cox/.

Research on Aging Act of 1974. Public Law 93–296. May 31, section 461.

Rettig, R. A. 1977. *Cancer Crusade: The Story of the National Cancer Act of 1971.* Princeton: Princeton University Press.

Rich, F. 2011. "Confessions of a Recovering Op-Ed Columnist." *New York Times.* March 13. http://www.nytimes.com/2011/03/13/opinion/13rich.html

Richardson, T. R. 1989. *The Century of the Child: Mental Health Hygiene and Social Policy in the United States and Canada.* Albany: State University of New York Press.

Rioch, D. M. 1985. "Recollections of Harry Stack Sullivan and the Development of His Interpersonal Psychiatry." *Psychiatry* 48:141–58.

Rioch, M. J. 1986 "Fifty Years at the Washington School of Psychiatry." *Psychiatry* 49:33–44.

Robinson, J. 2001. *Noble Conspirator: Florence S. Mahoney and the Rise of the National Institutes of Health.* Washington, D.C.: Francis Press.

Rockefeller, J. 2011. "Cable News 'Dumbing Down' the Discourse." http://theintel ligencer.net/page/content/id/549022/Sen—Rockefeller—Cable-News—Dumbing-Down—the-Discourse.html?nav=515.

Rogers, D. E. 1977. "The Challenge of Primary Care." *Daedalus* 106:81–103.

———. 1978. *American Medicine: Challenges for the 1980s.* Cambridge, Mass.: Ballinger.

Rosenberg, C. E. 1987. *The Care of Strangers: The Rise of America's Hospital System.* New York: Basic Books.

Rosenfield, A. 1998. "The View from the Dean's Office." *American Journal of Epidemiology* 147:201–2.

Rosenzweig, R. M., and B. Turlington. 1982. *The Research Universities and Their Patrons.* Berkeley: University of California Press.

Rowe, J. W. Forthcoming. *The Aging Society Project.* MacArthur Foundation.

Rowe, J. W., and R. L. Kahn. 1998. *Successful Aging.* New York: Pantheon Books.

Ruesch, J. 1978. *Langley Porter Institute and Psychiatry in Northern California: 1943–1975.* San Francisco: Friends of Langley Porter Institute.

Russo, F. 2010. "The Aging of America Portends Struggle, Empowerment and Sweeping Social Transformation." *Aging Today* 31:1–2.

Sankar, A., ed. 2011. *Generations.* Special Issue.

Sarkistan, C. A., et al. 2002. "Development, Reliability, and Validity of Expectations Regarding Aging (ERA-38) Survey." *Gerontologist* 42:534–42.

Satterfield, J. M., B. Spring, R. C. Brownson, E. J. Mullen, R. P. Newhouse, B. B. Walker, and E. P. Whitlock. 2009. "Toward a Transdisciplinary Model of Evidence-Based Practice." *Milbank Quarterly* 87 (2):368–90.

Saunders, P. A., J. R. Copeland, M. E. Dewey, I. A. Davidson, C. McWilliam, V. Sharma, and C. Sullivan. 1991. "Heavy Drinking as a Risk Factor for Depression and Dementia in Elderly Men." *British Journal of Psychiatry* 159 (August): 213–16.

Schachter-Shalomi, Z. 1995. *From Age-ing to Sage-ing.* New York: Warner.

Schafer, A. I., ed. 2009. *The Vanishing Physician-Scientist.* Ithaca: IRL/Cornell University Press.

Schechter, M. 1985. "Appendix A. Process and Perception: The Flavor and Framework of the Salzburg Seminar on Health, Productivity and Aging." In *Productive Aging: Enhancing Vitality in Later Life.* Edited by R. N. Butler and H. P. Gleason, 123–28. New York: Springer.

Schletter, T., and M. Valenti. 2010. "Environmental Threats to Healthy Aging: An Ecological Perspective." *Public Policy & Aging* 20:7.

Schoen, D. 1979. *Pat: A Biography of Daniel Patrick Moynihan.* New York: Harper and Row.

Schopenhauer, A. (1890) 1970. *Counsels and Maxims, Being the Second Part of Arthur Schopenhauer's Aphorismen zur Lebensweisheit.* Translated by T. B. Saunders. St. Clair Shores, Mich.: Scholarly Press.

Schwartz, J. 2011. "The Best-Laid Plans." *New York Times.* March 13.

Severo, R. "Mount Sinai Names a Chief Executive." 1983. *New York Times.* April 10. http://www.nytimes.com/1983/04/10/nyregion/mount-sinai-names-a-chief -executive.html.

Shabahangi, N., et al. 2009. "Some Observations on the Consequences of Forgetful- ness and Alzheimer's Disease." *Journal of Aging, Humanities and Arts* 3:38–52.

Shannon, J. A. 1967. "The Advancement of Medical Research: A Twenty-Year View of the Role of the National Institutes of Health." *Journal of Medical Education* 42:97–108.

———. 1971. "Medical Research: Some Aspects That Warrant Public Understand- ing." *New England Journal of Medicine* 284:75–80.

———. 1974. "Federal and Academic Relationships: The Biomedical Sciences 1974." *Proceedings of the National Academy of Science, USA* 71:3310–12.

Sheets, D. J., D. B. Bradley, and J. Hendricks, eds. 2006. *Enduring Questions in Gerontology.* New York: Springer.

Silverman, A. J., E. W. Busse, and R. H. Barnes. 1955. "Studies in the Processes of Aging: Electroencephalographic Findings in 400 Elderly Subjects." *Electroen- cephalography and Clinical Neurophysiology* 7 (February): 67–74.

Simon, A. 1948. "Alcohol. Geriatrics." *Review of Psychiatric Progress 1947,* 474–75.

———. 1971. "Community Mental Health Services." *California Medicine* 114:35–36.

———. 1984. "Some Observations of a Geropsychiatrist on the Value of House Calls." *Gerontologist* 24:458–64.

Simon, A., L. H. Margolis, J. E. Adams, and K. M. Bowman. 1951. "Unilateral and Bilateral Lobotomy." *Archives of Neurology and Psychiatry* 66 (4): 494–503.

Sinclair, M. 1989. "Betty Friedan Sheds Light on the 'Mystique' of Aging." *Or- lando Sentinel.* March 1. http://articles.orlandosentinel.com/1989-03- 01 /lifestyle/8903020261_1_older-women-betty-friedan-elderly-women.

Small, H., ed. 2002. *The Public Intellectual.* New York: Blackwell.

Smythe, C. M. 1967. "Developing Medical Schools." *Journal of Medical Education* 42:991–1004.

"Snapshots of the Premiere." 2010. http://info/toageornottoage.com/2010/02/
snapshots-of-the-premiere.

Sohm, P. 2007. *The Artist Grows Old: The Aging of Art and Artists in Italy,
1500–1800.* New Haven: Yale University Press.

Sokoloff, L. 2003. "Seymour S. Kety, 1915–2000." In *Biographical Memoirs.* Vol.
38. Washington, D.C.: National Academies Press. http://www.nap.edu/html
/biomems/skety.html.

Solberg, C. 1984. *Hubert Humphrey: A Biography.* New York: Norton.

"Space Aging." 1998. *New York Times.* October 29. http://www.nytimes.com
/1998/10/29/opinion/space-aging.html.

Squire, L. R., ed. 2011. *The History of Neuroscience in Autobiography.* Vol. 7. New
York: Oxford University Press.

Stadtman, V. A., ed. 1967. *The Centennial of the University of California, 1868–
1968: Psychiatry.* Berkeley: University of California.

Starr, P. 1982. *The Social Transformation of American Medicine.* New York: Basic
Books.

Stayner, L. 2008. "A Conversation with Jacob Brody." *Epidemiology* 19:756–59.

Stein, B. 2010. ""Ben Stein's Diary: Return from Sandpoint." *American Spectator.*
July 12. http://spectator.org/archives/2010/07/12/return-from-sandpoint.

Stek, M., D. J. Vinklers, R.L. Van der Mast, A.J.F. Beekman, and P.G.T. Westen-
dorp. 2006. "Natural History of Depression in the Oldest Old." *British Journal
of Psychiatry* 188:65–69.

Stetten, D., and W. T. Carrigan. 1984. *NIH: An Account of Research in Its Laboratories and Clinics.* Orlando: Academic Press.

Steunenberg, B., and E. Bohlmeijer. 2011. "Life Review Using Autobiographical
Retrieval: A Protocol for Training Depressed Residential Home Inhabitants
in Recalling Specific Personal Memories." In *Storying Later Life.* Edited by
G. Kenyon, E. Bohlmeijer, and W. L. Randall. New York: Oxford University Press.

Stossel, S. 1984. *Sarge: The Life and Times of Sargent Shriver.* Washington, D.C.:
Smithsonian Books.

Strickland, S. P. 1972. *Politics, Science, and Dread Disease: A Short History of
United States Medical Research Policy.* Cambridge: Harvard University Press.

Suppes, P. 1994. "Ernest Nagel: November 16, 1901–September 20, 1985." In *Biographical Memoirs.* Vol. 65. Washington, D.C.: National Academies Press.

Svanborg, A. 1985. "Biomedical and Environmental Influences on Aging." In *Productive Aging:Enhancing Vitality in Later Life.* Edited by R. N. Butler and
H. P. Gleason. New York: Springer.

Sykes, K., and K. Pillemer. 2009. "Gray and Green." *Generations* 33.

———. 2010. *Public Policy & Aging Report 20.*

Szasz, T. 1961. *The Myth of Mental Illness: Foundations of a Theory of Personal Conduct.* New York: Harper and Row.

Taggart, H. 1981. "Comment: Geriatric Medicine in the United States: A British View." *Age and Ageing* 10:69–72.

Tapper, J. 2010. "A Last Conversation with Dr. Robert Butler." *New York Times.* July 7.

Tavris, C., and E. Aronson. 2007. *Mistakes Were Made (but Not by Me).* Orlando: Harvest.

Thielens, W. 1958. "Some Comparisons of Entrants to Medical and Law School." *Journal of Legal Education* 11:153–68.

Thomas, L. 1972. *Aspects of Biomedical Science Policy.* Washington, D.C.: National Academies Press.

——. 1983. *Late Night Thoughts on Listening to Mahler's Ninth Symphony.* New York: Viking.

——. 1987. "What Doctors Don't Know." *New York Review of Books.* September 24. http://www.nybooks.com/articles/archives/1987/sep/24/what-doctors -dont-know/.

——. 1997. "The Hazards of Science." In *The Presence of Others.* Edited by A. A. Lunsford and J. J. Ruszkiewicz. New York: Bedford/St. Martin's.

Tornstam, L. 2005. *Gerotranscendence.* New York: Springer.

Townsend, C., ed. 1971. *Old Age: The Last Segregation (The Nader Report).* New York: Grossman.

Trattner, W. I. 1974. *From Poor Law to Welfare State.* New York: Free Press.

Turturro, A., W. W. Witt, S. Lewis, B. S. Hass, R. D. Lipman, and R. W. Hart. 1999. "Growth Curves and Survival Characteristics of the Animals Used in the Biomarkers of Aging Program." *Journals of Gerontology* 54: B492–501.

"Tutoring." n.d. http://www.ilcusa.org/pages/projects/ageism.php.

"2008 Macarthur Fellows—Diane Meier." 2008. http://www.macfound.org /fellows/805/.

United States Congress. 2001. *Congressional Record: Proceedings and Debates of the 107th Congress, First Session, Volume 147, Part 5.* Washington, D.C.: UNT Digital Library. http://digital.library.unt.edu/ark:/67531/metadc31060/.

United States Department of Health, Education, and Welfare (HEW). Office of the Surgeon General. 1979. *Healthy People: The Surgeon General's Report on Health Promotion and Disease Prevention.* Washington, D.C.: Government Printing Office.

United States Senate. 1971. *White House Conference on Aging: A Report to the Delegates from the Conference Sections and Special Concerns Sessions.* Senate Document 92-53. Washington, D.C.: Government Printing Office.

———. Special Committee on Aging, Subcommittee on Long-Term Care. 1971. *Trends in Long-Term Care*, Part 2. December 17, 1970. Washington, D.C.: Government Printing Office.

———. 1978. *The Graying of Nations.* Washington, D.C.: Government Printing Office.

University of California, San Francisco. 2010. "People: R. Langley Porter: 1870–1965." http://history.library.ucsf.edu/porter.html.

———. n.d. "Department of Psychiatry." http://psych.ucsf.edu/residency-programs.aspx?id=2032.

Van Doren, M. 1959. *Liberal Education.* 2d ed. Boston: Beacon Press.

Van Tassel, D. D., ed. 1979. *Aging, Death, and the Completion of Being.* Philadelphia: University of Pennsylvania Press.

Vella, M. 2008. "Can America Close the 'Innovation Gap'?" *Bloomberg Business Week.* http://www/businessweek.com/innovate/content/oct2008109...

Verbrugge, L. 1984. "Longer Life but Worsening Health? Trends in Health and Mortality of Middle-Aged and Older Persons." *Milbank Memorial Fund Quarterly* 62:475–519.

Veterans Health Administration. 2008. "Advanced Fellowships in Geriatrics: Program Announcement." Washington, D.C.: U.S. Department of Veterans Affairs.

Vickery, H. B. 1975. "Hans Thacher Clarke: December 27, 1887–October 21, 1972." In *Biographical Memoirs.* Vol. 46. Washington, D.C.: National Academies Press.

Viner, J. 1950. *A Modest Proposal for Some Stress on Scholarship in Graduate Training. Address Before the Graduate Convocation, Brown University, June 3, 1950.* Brown University Papers 24. Providence: Brown University.

von Preyss-Friedman, S. 2009. "Geriatrics Education and Training Experience in the United States." *Journal of the Korean Geriatrics Society* 13:1–6.

Walker, J. L. 1991. *Mobilizing Interest Groups in America: Patrons, Professions, and Social Movements.* Ann Arbor: University of Michigan Press.

Wallace, J. B. 1992. Reconsidering the Life Review: The Social Construction of Talk About the Past. *Gerontologist* 32:120–25.

Warner, H. R., et al. 2005. "Science Fact and the SENS Agenda." *EMBO Reports* 6:1006–8.

Warner, H. R., R. N. Butler, R. L. Sprott, and E. L. Schneider, eds. 1987. *Modern Biological Theories of Aging.* New York: Raven Press.

Warner, W. R. 2005. "Developing a Research Agenda in Biogerontology: Basic Mechanisms." *Scientific Aging Knowledge Environment* 44:33.

Webb, A. 2006. *Do Health and Longevity Create Wealth?* Alliance Policy Report for ILC-USA, ILC-France, and ILC-UK, 21–22.

Webster, J. D., E. T. Bohlmeijer, and G. J. Westerhof. 2010. "Mapping the Future of Reminiscence." *Research on Aging* 32:527–64.

Webster, J. D., and B. K. Haight, eds. 2002. *Critical Advances in Reminiscence Work: From Theory to Application.* New York: Springer.

Weinberg, J. 1995. "The Impact of Ageing upon the Need for Medical Beds: A Monte-Carlo Simulation. *Journal of Public Health Medicine* 17:290–96.

Weingarten, H. R. 1988. "Late Life Divorce and the Life Review." *Journal of Gerontological Social Work* 12:83–97.

Weissman, G. 2010. *Lewis Thomas.* Washington, D.C.: National Academies Press. http:www.nap.edu/readingroom.php?book=biomems&page=lthomas.html.

Wetle, T. F. 2010. "Remarks." Gerontological Society of America Memorial for Robert N. Butler, November 22.

Wheeler, D. P., and N. Giunta. 2009. "Promoting Productive Aging." *Health and Social Work* 34: 237–239.

Whitehouse, P. J., and D. George. 2008. *The Myth of Alzheimer's: What You Aren't Being Told About Today's Dreaded Diagnosis.* New York: St. Martin's Press.

Wildavsky, A. B. 1979. *Speaking Truth to Power: The Art and Craft of Policy Analysis.* Boston: Little, Brown.

Willard, H. W., and G. S. Ginsberg, eds. 2009. *Genomic and Personalized Medicine.* Academic Press.

Williams, T. F. 1986. Interview by L. Keegan. [Audio Tape Recording]. "NIA's T. Franklin Williams." Provider (May): 52–55. http://www.biomedsearch.com/nih/interview-with-Robert-Butler-Interview/6832606.html.

Wilson, D. L. 1968. "The Ambulatory Clinic in a Teaching Hospital." *Canadian Medical Association Journal* 98: 812–14.

Wilson, J. T. 1983. *Academic Science, Higher Education, and the Federal Government: 1950–1983.* Chicago: University of Chicago Press.

Wilson, M. P., and C. P. McLaughlin. 1984. *Leadership and Management in Academic Medicine.* San Francisco: Jossey-Bass.

Winnicott, D. W. 1971. *Playing and Reality.* London: Tavistock.

Woo, B. 2006. "Primary Care—The Best Job in Medicine?" *New England Journal of Medicine* 355:864–66.

Wood, D. 2008. "Life Review: The Benefits of Recording Your 'Autobiography.' " *healthlibrary.* http://healthlibrary.epnet.com/GetContent.aspx?token=a4c1f00b-d245–44f2-a90e-20b047.

Woodward, K. M. 1986. "Reminiscence and Life Review." In *What Does It Mean to Grow Old.* Edited by T. R. Cole and S. Gadow, 135–61. Durham: Duke University Press.

———. 1997. *Telling Stories: Aging, Reminiscence, and the Life Review.* Berkeley: University of California, Doreen B. Townsend Center for the Humanities.

———. 2002. "Against Wisdom: The Social Politics of Anger and Aging." *Cultural Critique* 51:186–216.

Woolf, S. H. 2008. "The Meaning of Translational Research and Why It Matters." *Journal of the American Medical Association* 299:211–13.

Yoshikawa, T. T. 2006a. "Paul Beeson, MD: Today's Sir William Osler." *Journal of the American Geriatric Society* 54 (11):1639–40.

———. 2006b. "Remembering Paul Beeson, MD, 1908–2006." *AGS News*, 37.

Zelewski, S. R., and B. A. Butrica. 2007. "Are We Taking Full Advantage of Older Adults' Potential?" Perspectives on Productive Aging. *Urban Institute* 9:1–8.

INDEX

p x B — should try "offers a keen approach to addressing older
people's resources and resilience while attending to decrease and
challenges of later life"
— B confrontational & replace stereotypes with images of accorded
older individuals everywhere dignity and respect
xv "AGISM REMAINS ENDEMIC" — there was few ways to agony than
& Early in his professional career convened —
declining professional career convened.
B's 3 quotes — ARISTOTLE, CONFUCIUS, MOUCHAM.

LAST THOUGHTS used MONTAIGNE, CAMUS, BECKETT, JOHN BAYLEY.
p16 B "no church goer" — but was torn from Theology,
p22 Value of renewal "... in des Kaugh, then confusing well
p34 Burton (in 1959 speech) — exciting prevalent attitudes — the older
FEEBLE UNINTERESTING / HE AWAITS HIS DEATH) A
BURDEN to SOCIETY, to HIS FAMILY AND TO HIMSELF
— enjoying "having there love" He
1974 Senate Special Cttee on Aging
US — Future in Public policy.
p77 His 3 arms,
GSA founded 1945.
"unaffiliated with any faith congregation"
p81 B (1958)
p84 its original foundation of Ogon (1968)
why SUBSIDE — fd 1976 PULITZER PRIZES (when B was 49)
p158 USA shown of roots in Genetics — no duplo prior to 1988 — pioneer,
GOZZ OLD, centered OK deal.
p116 B (1979) need for US to "recognize the new found resources of
strength and capability" — loyalty a Ted Myseld. Approach B to
p122 Pregnancy / HOOVER SIGN — loyalty a Ted Myseld.
the change!
B (p126) wrote extensively sympathetic views on aging.
p131 1983 SALZBURG SEMINAR (50 valuing)
p148 1987 — visited Japan. 1990 — will help of all US govt —
established US branch of INTERNATIONAL LONGEVITY CENTRE / — funded in excess
p p26 M by "ATLANTIC PHILANTHROPIES" — fell 100 T 130 gate
further,
p136 "ADVOCATES OF ANTI-AGEING MEDICINES CREATED KEX CLADDED GERONTOLOGISTS"